INTERPRETING
THE
MEDICAL
LITERATURE

Jan '94

To Rob —
Happy interpreting —

Steve

INTERPRETING THE MEDICAL LITERATURE

THIRD EDITION

Stephen H. Gehlbach, M.D., M.P.H.

Dean and Professor, School of Public Health
University of Massachusetts
Amherst, Massachusetts

McGRAW-HILL, INC.
Health Professions Division

New York   St. Louis   San Francisco   Auckland   Bogotá   Caracas
Lisbon   London   Madrid   Mexico   Milan   Montreal   New Delhi
Paris   San Juan   Singapore   Sydney   Tokyo   Toronto

INTERPRETING THE MEDICAL LITERATURE

1234567890 DOCDOC 98765432

ISBN 0-07-105451-0

This book was set in Times Roman by Northeastern Graphic Services, Inc.
The editors were Gail Gavert and Muza Navrozov.
The production supervisor was Richard Ruzycka.
The cover and text were designed by José Fonfrias.
The index was prepared by Philip James.
R.R. Donnelley & Sons Company was printer and binder.

Library of Congress Cataloging-in-Publication Data

Gehlbach, Stephen H.
    Interpreting the medical literature / Stephen H. Gehlbach.
    — 3rd ed.
        p.   cm.
    Includes bibliographical references and index.
    ISBN 0-07-105451-0
    1. Medical literature.   2. Medicine—Research.   3. Epidemiology-
-Terminology.   I. Title.
    [DNLM: 1. Epidemiology—terminology.   2. Periodicals.
3. Research—methods.   W 20.5 G311i]
RM111.6.G43   1993
610.72—dc20
DNLM/DLC
for Library of Congress   92–49250
                                                              CIP

CONTENTS

Preface . . . . *ix*

CHAPTER ONE

TASTING AN ARTICLE 1

Validity *3*
Reasons to Read *4*
The Bones of an Article *6*
Approaching an Article *9*

CHAPTER TWO

STUDY DESIGN:
GENERAL CONSIDERATIONS 14

Descriptive Studies *15*
Explanatory Studies *18*
More Confusing Terminology *27*
Summary *32*

CHAPTER THREE

STUDY DESIGN:
THE CASE-CONTROL APPROACH 34

Advantages of the Case-Control Design *35*
Problems of Case-Control Designs *36*
Summary *51*

CHAPTER FOUR

STUDY DESIGN:
THE CROSS-SECTIONAL
AND FOLLOW-UP APPROACHES 55

Cross-Sectional Designs *57*
Follow-up Studies *67*
Summary *74*

CHAPTER FIVE

STUDY DESIGN:
THE EXPERIMENTAL APPROACH 78

Subjects: Who Gets in *79*
Controls: Their Presence and Comparability *87*
The Intervention or Treatment *93*
Allocation: Subject Assignment *99*
Attrition *104*
End Points *106*
Summary *107*

CHAPTER SIX

MAKING MEASUREMENTS 111

Reliability and Validity *112*
Variability of the Unsystematic Sort *113*
Systematic Error *116*
Controlling Measurement Error *122*
Summary *124*

CHAPTER SEVEN

INTERPRETATION: DISTRIBUTIONS,
AVERAGES, AND THE NORMAL 127

Frequency Distributions *128*
Measures of Central Tendency *130*
Indicators of Variability *132*
Normality *134*
Regression to the Mean *140*
Summary *143*

CHAPTER EIGHT

INTERPRETATION: STATISTICAL SIGNIFICANCE 145

Inference *146*
Sampling Variability *147*
The Null Hypothesis and Statistical Significance *148*
Some Problems of Statistical Significance *149*
Beta Errors and Statistical Power *154*
Confidence Intervals *156*
Testing for Statistical Significance May Be Irrelevant *157*
Summary *159*

CHAPTER NINE

INTERPRETATION: SOME STATISTICAL TESTS 161

Tests for Continuous Data *166*
Correlation *169*
Regression *171*
Summary *176*

CHAPTER TEN

INTERPRETATION: SENSITIVITY, SPECIFICITY, AND PREDICTIVE VALUE 178

Prevalence *184*
Making Choices *187*
Multiple Tests *188*
Spectrum *193*
Standards *194*
Cost Considerations *196*
Summary *198*

CHAPTER ELEVEN

INTERPRETATION: RISK 201

Statements of Risk *202*
Relative Risk *203*
Relative Risk and Study Design *204*

Attributable Risk *209*
Balancing Risks *210*
Summary *212*

CHAPTER TWELVE
INTERPRETATION: CAUSES .214
Confounding *215*
Dealing with Confounding *218*
Making Associations into Causes *223*
Summary *229*

CHAPTER THIRTEEN
CASE SERIES, EDITORIALS,
AND REVIEWS 231
Case Series *232*
Editorials and Letters to the Editor *239*
Reviews *243*
Summary *249*

CHAPTER FOURTEEN
A FINAL WORD 252
Clarity *253*
Apologies, Tentative Conclusions, Self-Criticism, and the Like *255*
The Final Word *256*
Summary *258*

Index 259

PREFACE

$\mathcal{T}$he purpose of this book is to provide clinicians with an approach to reading and understanding research articles that appear in medical journals. Although it is not a text of epidemiology, it is based on principles of that discipline and on a way of thinking that is epidemiological. The terms used in discussing concepts will come primarily from epidemiology rather than from the social sciences research tradition. Most medical readers will already have some familiarity with jargon, such as "case-control and cohort studies," "sensitivity and specificity," and "relative risk." An understanding of these terms is essential to the comprehension of medical articles, and they are discussed in modest detail; but because the book is intended as a guide for clinicians—people who need to make practical use of medical literature—extensive forays into epidemiology's semantic jungle will be avoided. Some depth will be sacrificed for the sake of brevity. The goal is to acquire skill with a few fundamental analytical tools and avoid becoming mired in complexity.

The book is intended for several levels of clinical learners. It is hoped that medical students, who are beginning to form reading habits, will benefit from an early exposure to the concepts of adequate study design, appropriate sample selection, and use of statistical inference. More seasoned clinicians should become more comfortable with old stumbling blocks, such as "selection bias" and "the null hypothesis."

Throughout the book, I have attempted to update examples. Some that seem no longer to hold current interest have been dropped. Others, despite having been published some years ago, are still timely; heart disease, urinary tract infection, and postpartum depression have not gone out of fashion. A few examples, though somewhat dated, illustrate points so nicely it is difficult to displace them. Readers comparing this with previous editions will certainly notice the increased prevalence of illustrations related to HIV/AIDS, a reflection of the importance of the epidemic and the volume of literature the problem has spawned. I have also attempted some reorganization within chapters and some rewriting to improve clarity.

Because clinical applicability and relevance are major goals, I have continued to use illustrations that come from published articles. The sparkle of authenticity that this provides is somewhat tarnished by the appearance of being critical toward colleagues. None of the critiques of examples used in this book is intended to be disparaging of the authors. Conducting good clinical research is a formidable task. There is substantial risk in exposing one's work to the harsh light of publication. Because of the difficulties inherent in studying and documenting the behavior of humans, it is a rare study indeed that is beyond fault. I think the advantages of using published articles exceed the liabilities. Real examples give readers the opportunity to examine primary sources for themselves, practice their analytical skills, and formulate dissenting views.

A final admonition: As with developing clinical skills, such as examining tympanic membranes or listening for heart murmurs, acquiring proficiency in reading the medical literature requires practice. Most of the principles discussed in this book will appear simple and are reasonably straightforward—but that is not to say that their application will come easily to everyone. Facility and comfort will come only through practice. Like visualizing the fundus of the eye, it is not difficult once you get the hang of it, but it takes work to develop and maintain the skill.

The assistance of colleagues, among them Dave Hosmer, deserves special mention. I am particularly indebted to Tom Newman, who gave the second edition a thorough going-over and provided many useful suggestions. Sandy Wake and Hilary Gehlbach provided great help in assembling this third edition.

INTERPRETING THE MEDICAL LITERATURE

CHAPTER ONE

TASTING AN ARTICLE

Some books are to be tasted, others to be swallowed, and some few to be chewed and digested.

FRANCIS BACON

$\mathcal{K}$eeping up with the medical literature is a strenuous proposition. The stacks of unread journals that collect on desks and in filing cabinets during medical school and residency training only grow larger. The number of textbooks, yearbooks, newsletters, and specialty journals swells, while the time to read them shrinks. Yet we are pressed to keep current from several sides. Most of us are taught early in medical training that to be a good physician one must keep abreast of the latest in clinical syndromes, novel diagnostic tests, and innovative treatments. We need to learn which environmental carcinogens to avoid and how to improve our understanding of the causes of heart disease. Specialty boards and medical societies reinforce this concept by requiring documentation of continuing education for certification and for society membership. Some recertification plans specifically call for examinations based on information from the current literature.

Patients also expect informed physicians. Like their doctors, they are beset with medical facts and fiction from radio, television, and the popular press. Whether they read the *New York Times* or a supermarket tabloid, they are likely to be getting information that is at least in part based on reports from the medical literature. Patients want to

1

know about their risk of contracting Lyme disease when they visit Connecticut, whether their headaches deserve a CT scan, or if Dr. Nocal's water-only diet really works.

Even though the spirit may be willing, the eyes grow weak, and the task of sorting through the mounds of published material seems a losing affair. Some remedy would appear to come from the many secondary sources that are available. Medical textbooks, special review journals, newsletters, and audio cassettes supply synthesized information on current topics. One can easily read the collected opinions of experts about everything from ankylosing spondylitis to tropical zoonoses from one of several excellent textbooks, or listen to a learned colleague discuss lead poisoning while driving to work, thanks to the wonders of magnetic tape. Secondary sources are an efficient way to gather information and circumvent the painful process of trying to master the complicated presentation of data in primary sources. Experts have problems like the rest of us. Sometimes their subjective selves get the upper hand and cast controversy into fact. Opinions and biased reading can become standard knowledge. That should not surprise us, since many studies are open to differing interpretation. It does mean, however, that while texts and reviews are useful, we cannot depend entirely on secondary sources for our information. We need to be able to evaluate a primary research article ourselves and judge its value.

Finding time to do this reading is not the only challenge. Articles describing clinical studies have become increasingly sophisticated. Not only has the complexity of the information presented increased, the methods used to obtain and interpret data have become correspondingly complex. Clinical studies now utilize "stratified sampling techniques," "randomized double-blind crossover designs," and a multitude of semicomprehensible techniques for statistical analysis. Understanding the nuances of these methodologies is every bit as demanding as keeping up with the side effects of the latest pharmacological agents or the newest discoveries of immune-cell function.

The purpose of this book is to give practical aid to the beleaguered clinician. This chapter will offer advice on general approaches to reading articles—on exercising our powers of selectivity and efficiency. As Francis Bacon suggested some 400 years ago, much of the written material that comes our way deserves only a perfunctory taste, with relatively few articles meriting full digestion.

Once we have developed some rules for making initial decisions about which articles to read and have gained an overall sense of what they are about, we can proceed with more detailed critical review. Chapters will be devoted to exploring the design of studies, classifying methodologies, and learning about their basic strengths and weaknesses. The problems encountered in making measurements and collecting data in a satisfactory manner will be a second concern; we will examine observer and subject biases. Finally, ways in which data are analyzed and interpreted will be discussed.

The goal of all this will be to arrive at an interpretation we can call our own. We will balance the strengths and flaws uncovered in an article and come up with an independent assessment of whether the author's message rings true—whether in the final analysis acupuncture successfully reduces pain or treating mild hypertension lowers morbidity from stroke. The bottom line is validity. Are the results believable? Do they represent the truth? Are they applicable to our practice? Will the patients we see and treat respond in the same way as those described in the study? Does the paper really support its claims?

VALIDITY

The concept of validity is central to the critical analysis of the medical literature. We will continue to encounter it in several forms throughout the book. Two types of validity will be of concern. The first relates to the internal structure of the study. In their discussion of experimental designs, Campbell and Stanley call it *internal validity*.[1] They mean that within the confines of the study, results appear to be accurate, the methods and analysis used bear up under scrutiny, and the interpretation of the investigators appears supported. For the particular subjects evaluated, hydrochlorothiazide appears to be better than placebo in reducing high blood pressure, smokers seem to experience more chronic lung disease than nonsmokers, or obstetrical units with fetal-monitoring devices have lower rates of perinatal problems. Truth is told.

There is another type of validity that we will discuss. Called *external validity* by the social scientists,[1] it is more commonly thought of by medical people as generalizability. Generalizability is terribly important to clinicians. It has to do with whether conclusions (if internally valid) can be applied to the reader's setting or practice. We will return to it in later chapters.

REASONS TO READ

I have already alluded to the general goal of keeping current as a reason for reading journals. Medical journals offer more than reports of recent information on tests, treatments, and concepts of etiology. They provide a fascinating potpourri of opinion, philosophy, argument, gossip, history, theory, and advice. I have mentioned the topical review articles that condense up-to-date thoughts on the treatment of congestive heart failure or use of ultrasound technology. Individual authors may be responsible for these reports or, occasionally, expert committees may publish their consensus on a controversial topic such as the treatment of febrile seizures or the prophylactic use of antibiotics in hospitals. Practical hints, such as diagnosing scabies in the office or setting up pension plans for employees, are features of some journals. Comments published as letters to the journal and sage remarks made by the editors can make engaging and informative reading. These are especially valuable when they offer informed critiques of research articles or when authors debate the results of research in an open forum. There are pieces that discuss aspects of the history of the profession (such as a review of smallpox immunization in early Boston), views from other parts of the medical world, or philosophical pieces on the wonders and frailties of our medical system.

That is a splendid array of offerings, and I have not mentioned the book reviews, employment opportunities, and news of professional organizations. Any part of this list makes legitimate reading, but none falls into the category of primary research, which is the meat for our discussion. Among the new ideas and information available to readers are the choices listed in Table 1-1. They span a spectrum—from learning about Lyme disease and "environmental illness" to sharing the collective experiences of Florida physicians with malpractice claims.

This rich smorgasbord is worth noting, since reasons for picking up a journal will vary. The approach one takes in reading an article

• TABLE 1-1 •	
Some reasons for reading medical articles	
Read to find out about:	**For example:**
New health problems	Environmental illness
	Cumulative trauma disorders
New presentation or manifestations of diseases	Tuberculosis in AIDS patients
Extent and natural history of diseases	Prevalence of HIV among university students
	Sequelae of bacterial meningitis in children
Accuracy of diagnostic procedures	Screening for alcohol abuse
	Ruling out myocardial infarction
New treatments or programs	Treatment of traveler's diarrrhea
	Effectiveness of a home health care team
Adverse effects of medical care	Benzodiazepines and accidental injury
	Hospital characteristics and adverse events
Causes (and non-causes) and predictors of disease	Cancer risk from passive smoking
	Video display terminals and abortion
Experience of others	Ultrasound in recurrent abdominal pain
	Medical malpractice experience of physicians

depends very much on the intent at the outset. Reading to review the pathophysiology of Rocky Mountain spotted fever or to learn what an expert committee thinks is the proper way to work up a urinary tract infection is a different process from assessing the validity of a report linking artificial sweeteners to bladder cancer or the results of a study demonstrating the benefits of a new antacid for treating peptic ulcers. Deciding in advance what you wish to obtain from the journal is the first step to more efficient reading.

Understanding the framework of articles also facilitates efficient reading. Mortimer J. Adler has produced an entire volume on how to read a book.[2] In it, he emphasizes that effective reading requires identifying and understanding the structure or components of a work. That, he states, contributes to the "intelligibility of the whole." Adler's advice on reading books has parallels for the reader of medical journals. His medical metaphor to approaching a great book has an irresistible message for clinicians:

> Every book has a skeleton hidden between its boards. Your job is to find it. A book comes to you with flesh on its bare bones and clothes over its flesh. It is all dressed up. I am not asking you to be impolite or cruel. You do not have to undress it or tear the flesh off its limbs to get at the firm structure that underlies the soft. But you must read the book with x-ray eyes, for it is an essential part of your first apprehension of any book to grasp its structure.[2]

THE BONES OF AN ARTICLE

Most articles that deliver new information to readers share a basic structural plan. The six main sections outlined in Table 1-2 are usually present.

The *summary* or *abstract* should present a concise statement of the goal or hypothesis of the study, a word or two about how the endeavor was undertaken, highlights of the results, and a concluding thought that puts it all into perspective. To facilitate this, many journals have introduced "structured abstracts."[3] While the formats for these vary from journal to journal, they generally organize information by useful headings such as "Study Objective," "Design," "Results," etc. Not only do structured abstracts provide readers with a useful guide but they also encourage authors to attend to details about method that are sometimes overlooked.* Readers should be able to glean a reasonable sense of the contents of a journal by flipping past the antacid advertisements and scanning just the abstracts. One could do worse than be a nibbler of abstracts. One sometimes needs to do better, however. Abstracts provide a useful taste of the contents of the study, but they are rarely sufficient to make a meal in themselves. Because of the need

---

*Not everyone agrees that structured abstracts are a great advance. Differing views are available for those interested in the topic.[4-7]

• Table 1-2 •	
The basic structure of an article	
Section:	**Look for the following:**
Abstract/Summary	Overview or summary of the work Highlights of results General statement of significance
Introduction	Background information: history, pathophysiology, clinical presentation Review of the work of others Rationale for present study
Methods/Materials & Methods/ Patients & Methods	Study design Subject selection procedures Methods of measurement Description of analytic techniques
Results	What happened? Graphics—tables, charts, figures—that summarize findings
Discussion/Comment/Conclusion	Meaning, significance of work Critique of study: discussion of limitations as well as strengths, further analysis Comparison with work of others Disclaimers, equivocation, apologies, chest thumping, speculation, instruction, fantasy, and so on
References/Bibliography	Evidence that work of others has been considered Leads to further exploration of the subject

to be concise, abstracts select only the highlights of a paper. They are also, quite understandably, an author's attempt to put his best foot forward. Sometimes the author's summary of the article contains more wish than reality and presents a distorted view of the work that follows. Deception is probably not intended, but vigorous condensation can impart false emphasis.

The *introduction* section of the paper usually provides background information on the topic to be addressed, as well as rationale for why the authors undertook the adventure. Sometimes the introduction will offer an extended review of other literature surrounding the topic. When well done, this provides readers with a nourishing appetizer before they undertake the main course of the paper; it may, in itself, make the reading worthwhile.

The next section describes the *methodology* of the study. It is labeled "Materials and Methods," "Patients and Methods," or some other variation on that theme. It details the patient populations studied, study designs utilized, and data collection techniques employed; it describes in more detail than many of us care to know the analytical and evaluative procedures used in the course of the study. This is the section that most readers skip. In fact, it is the section that some journals relegate to small print. It is also the section to which we will devote much of our analytical energy and to which we will return repeatedly in future chapters.

The *results* section, quite logically, presents the information obtained from the execution of the study. Results are usually found both in the text and in accompanying tables, charts, graphs, and figures. Analysis and some interpretation of the data are also presented in the results section. Like the methods section, the results section represents an essential part of the main bill of fare and will be discussed at considerable length.

An interesting mix of ingredients can go into fashioning the *discussion* of an article. A further analysis of the results may be accomplished; results and conclusions of other studies may be compared and contrasted; the author may offer apologies for oversights and transgressions or build a case to strengthen and support results. The discussion section is usually the most speculative and often the most interesting reading in the medical paper. Authors may review and comment upon other studies related to their own and usually try to place the results in perspective. It can make especially entertaining reading if the author's interpretation of the work is quite different from your own.

A list of *references* or a bibliography usually finishes off an article. Little more need be said about the references except that they are most conspicuous in their absence. Few authors are writing on topics so novel that some thought and other research has not gone on before. The list of references gives a reader a clue to how diligently authors have researched and reviewed the experience of other workers. An extensive, well-done bibliography that provides easy access to a wide selection of articles on a topic can save hours of hunting through library reference works and is sometimes the saving grace of an otherwise lackluster journal article.

Having a firm idea of what you wish to gain from reading a journal and knowing how to utilize the framework of an article to best advantage gets you off to a proper start. With this background, a few rules for sampling the literature are needed.

APPROACHING AN ARTICLE

Read only what is interesting and useful

Whether the cause is overzealous toilet training or an oppressive system of early education, most of us have acquired a disquieting degree of compulsive behavior by the time we reach medical school or clinical practice. This trait is not without value. It helps us master the many facts that form the foundation of our clinical practice and drives us to persist in attacking a patient's ketoacidosis at 2 o'clock in the morning. However, compulsiveness has its liabilities as well. Confronted with a burgeoning pile of medical journals, we cannot bear the thought that any of the information packaged within those glossy pages should go unlearned. We wait for that magical time when we can sit down and plow through it. That day never arrives, and our guilt grows proportionally with the stack, diminishing only occasionally when a few spare hours enable us to prune the pile by one or two or when a housekeeping purge assigns it all irrevocably to the attic or trash bin. Mental health demands that we become more selective readers. Rather than trying to devour every last article, we need to develop tactics for sampling journals and consuming only those articles that are most nutritious.

Our first taste of an article should have a selective purpose. What is the article about? Is it a topic of interest? Is the information likely to be useful? If an article is not of interest, do not read it! There is plenty of information overloading our synapses as it is. There is no point in burdening the system with information that will not be used. It takes up time and space and probably will not be retained. Of course there is a risk in making choices. The case report dismissed as unworthy after a quick look may well be just like a case that strolls into your office next Friday or becomes the topic of a discussion at grand rounds. So be it. Selective reading is an even greater problem for students, who must read omnivorously to define their areas of interest and for whom examinations and interrogating attending physicians are ever-present incentives to acquire information. It is probably at this stage in the development of a medical career that bad reading habits develop and the sense of duty to read indiscriminately becomes entrenched. The solution to the problem is simple in concept and difficult in execution.

1. Scan the table of contents and decide what each article is about.

2. Select articles to be pursued in greater detail and bypass those that are not of interest. (The faint of heart who are reluctant to make this decision on the basis of a title alone may consult the abstract.)

3. Do not equivocate. Do not accumulate a pile of maybes. Articles that might be useful in the future but are of little interest now usually do not get read. All of us like to hedge our bets against that time when we will encounter that rare new genetic syndrome or want to know how to treat a patient with glycogen storage disease, but medical libraries are full of just such advice. Pursue such information when the special need arises.

Scan the article to gain a quick overview

An important corollary to selective reading is to hold back the initial impulse to bite right into an article. Step back for a brief, circumspect view of the whole. You may be surprised at what you discover. Finding page after page of uninterrupted, double-column print may permanently dampen your enthusiasm or relegate the piece to a day when you really do have more time to spend. A quick flip through may tell you that the technical complexity of the article is more than you are prepared to take on. Unintelligible jargon or complicated mathematical formulas may suggest that your reading time would be more profitably spent elsewhere. You may discover on this quick perusal that an article you thought would offer practical clinical tidbits is actually a report of highly specialized laboratory work—a piece listed in the contents as "Cow's Milk Allergy" turns out to report on "the production of a lymphokine, the leukocyte-migration-inhibition factor, by peripheral blood lymphocytes in response to an in vitro challenge with bovine beta-lactoglobulin"[8]—or that an article from which you anticipated exciting new information is only a revival of some well-known old facts. Look over the graphs and tables. These are particularly useful in giving a perspective, since they are usually carefully selected by authors to summarize the main messages of the piece (worth more than many thousand words, as they say).

Scanning gives the reader a sense of the structure of an article, a perspective in which to organize thoughts. Many articles will, within the basic framework already described, offer subheadings that facilitate this structuring process. Scan them. A competent author, as Adler suggests, has organized the architecture of a work to be a functional, intelligible guide to the whole.

Concentrate on the methods section

Once one decides that an article is worth reading and one's appetite has not been dulled by the quick scan, a new approach is needed. Most readers begin and end with the abstract. Those with the fortitude to take on more of the article generally proceed to the introduction, pale at the prospect of reading the small print in the methods section, and skip it. Sometimes they also pass over tedious presentations of results in favor of finding out what happens at the end. Since the author usually rehashes the results and offers an overall interpretation of the study in the discussion section, heading straight for the last section seems an economical way to proceed.

Fitzgerald[9] has supplied evidence that "methods" are often not favored fare. During ward rounds, she passed out an article on diabetic retinopathy to a group of 11 medical students and interns. They were instructed to read the paper and two companion articles carefully for discussion at a subsequent rounds. As a test of critical reading savvy, Fitzgerald substituted for the methods section of the paper a comparable section from an entirely different article. Only one of the eight learners who read the paper noticed the substitution.

One purpose of this book is to retrain clinicians to focus on the methodology. Read the methods section first. Here is the substance of the research. Any new information, no matter how enthusiastically discussed or fervently endorsed, is only as useful as the methods and results are sound. Once we train ourselves to look critically at articles, the discussion sections in many will become superfluous. The design or analysis in an article may be so deficient that no amount of explanation, extrapolation, or apology on the part of the author can set it right. In this case, we have saved reading time by not pursuing the discussion of a study that is so marred that any conclusions drawn would lack validity.

Reserve the right of final judgment

One last and very important principle remains. The ultimate interpretation and decision about the value of an article rests with the reader. Too frequently, clinicians are cowed by the power of the printed word. After all, the author has reviewed the literature, designed and executed the study, and presented a convincing array of results. Who are we to quibble with the interpretation? It is only reasonable to defer to the experts. That is why reading only the introduction and discussion sections of the paper seems so efficient—a little background followed by an erudite discussion of the results.

Do not be fooled! We have every right to pin our own interpretation on the results. The burden of proof is upon the authors to convince us that they are right. The whole purpose of the exercise of critical reading is to provide clinicians with skills to analyze the article and make an independent assessment of whether it is worthy. It is a matter of educating the palate.

But a word of caution! Because it is much easier to reject an article as unsound than to give it unqualified praise, it is easy to become cynical about interpreting medical articles. If we look hard and long enough, we are bound to find some blemishes in the best of reported studies. For the reader, the task is to acknowledge human imperfection and decide whether, given the limitations of almost any study, the net effect of the work is valid and useful. In the final analysis, can we believe the results? Is the work applicable to our clinic operation and the kinds of patients we see?

Bear in mind through the next chapters that, although the pitfalls associated with designing and executing medical studies seem numerous and the apparent defects in published works many, there is much valuable information waiting to be chewed and digested.

REFERENCES

1. Campbell DT, Stanley JC: *Experimental and Quasi-experimental Designs for Research*. Chicago, Rand McNally, 1966.
2. Adler MJ: *How to Read a Book: The Art of Getting a Liberal Education*. New York, Simon & Schuster, 1940.
3. Haynes RB, Mulrow CD, Huth EJ, et al: More informative abstracts revisited. *Ann Intern Med* 113:69, 1990.
4. Heller MB: *Structured abstracts: A modest dissent. J Clin Epidemiol* 44:739, 1991.
5. Naylor CD, Williams JI, Guyatt G: Structured abstracts of proposals for clinical and epidemiological studies. *J Clin Epidemiol* 44:731, 1991.
6. Naylor CD, Williams JI, Guyatt G: Structured abstracts versus unstructured abstractions. *J Clin Epidemiol* 44:741, 1991.
7. Spitzer WO: The structured sonnet. *J Clin Epidemiol* 44:729, 1991.
8. Ashkenazi A, Levin S, Idar D, et al: In vitro cell-mediated immunologic assay for cow's milk allergy. *Pediatrics* 65:399, 1980.
9. Fitzgerald FT: From Galen to Xerox: The authoritarian reference in medicine. *Ann Intern Med* 96:245, 1982.

CHAPTER TWO

STUDY DESIGN: GENERAL CONSIDERATIONS

I'll no more on't: it hath made me mad.

HAMLET, *Act III, Scene I*

*A*lthough Hamlet may not have been specifically discussing his feelings on the taxonomy of study designs, he could well have been. Sorting through the maze of terms that are commonly employed to describe the design of studies could totter the stablest mind or flutter the stoutest heart. We are likely to encounter references to retrospective and prospective studies, prevalence, case-control and cohort studies, follow-up, and cross-sectional and trohoc studies. Along with longitudinal studies and incidence studies, there are experimental studies and clinical trials. We even get combinations such as retrospective cohort studies. The list goes on, but at this point most readers are ready to throw their hands skyward in irrevocable despair. How did we arrive at such a confusing state of affairs and what can a relatively reasonable soul expect to gain from making some sense of the taxonomy of study design?

Epidemiologists are probably most to blame for the glut of terminology. As methodologists they are rightfully concerned with precise definitions of the tools of their trade. Unfortunately, no one in the union seems able to accept the definitions of other members, and the neologisms have sprouted. One article in an epidemiology journal describes and discusses 23 definitions of the word "epidemiology."[1] Alas, as is the case with new cars and remedies for colds, the proliferation of terms describing study designs suggests that none is entirely satisfactory.

Although it is tempting for the clinician to leave this semantic tangle to those who enjoy it, there are several principles about study design that the intelligent reader needs to master. The trick is to keep the forest in view without floundering in the foliage. Identifying the structure of a study gives the reader a jump in assessing the validity of an article. Just as facts about the make and model of an automobile suggest predictive features about its gas mileage, repair record, and comfort, the facts about a study provide insight about strengths to be anticipated and weaknesses to probe for.

Let us begin with an overview to put the elements of study design into perspective. For purposes of the discussion we will not haggle about terminology. The goal is to get at the concepts that underlie designs. Table 2-1 supplies a schematic of the basic designs into which most medical studies fall. A large number of reports in the literature can be designated as descriptive, as seen on the left-hand side of the table.

DESCRIPTIVE STUDIES

As the term suggests, descriptive articles serve chiefly to record events, observations, and activities. They do not provide detailed explanations of the causes of disease or offer the kind of evidence we need to evaluate the efficacy of new treatments. They are, however, invaluable documentaries that, once filed, may lead to exciting discoveries. At its least complicated, a descriptive study is a report of a case or a small series of cases that an observer feels should be brought to the attention of colleagues. An account of an unusual episode of poisoning or an atypical rash developing after administration of a new medication are examples of descriptive studies at their simplest. These reports alert clinicians about possible drug side effects, unusual complications of illnesses, or surprising presentations of diseases. Caution must always be exercised in interpreting a single report or series of cases, since it

• **Table 2-1** •
Basic study designs

EXPLANATORY

Examine etiology, cause, efficacy, using the strategy of comparisons

DESCRIPTIVE

Document and communicate experience: share ideas, programs, treatments, unusual events, and observations

Begin search for explanations

Examples:

Case report or series
- Rash developing during drug treatment
- Cluster of cases of Kaposi's sarcoma

Clinical series
- Treatment of 50 snakebite victims

Population
- Prevalence of HIV in military recruits
- Community survey of needs of elderly

Program or course
- Course on sexuality for medical students

EXPERIMENTAL

Evaluate efficacy of therapeutic, educational, administrative interventions

Investigator controls allocation

Examples:

Clinical trial
- Comparison of two antidepressant drugs
- Surgical vs. medical management of angina

Educational intervention
- Self-instruction vs. lecture on anemia

Health-care trial
- Nurse practitioner vs. physician care

OBSERVATIONAL

Seek causes, etiologies, predictors, better diagnosis

Investigator observes nature

Examples:

Case-control
- Diets of toxemic vs. nontoxemic patients

Follow-up
- Development of renal complications in school-girls with bacteriuria

Cross-sectional
- Prediction of bacteremia in febrile children

is not always clear that the unusual rash or ringing in the ears reported by the patient who has been given a new antibiotic is related to the drug; however, the observations first noted in descriptive studies often lead to further, confirmatory work that produces important findings.

Case reports have been around for a long time. Consider William Heberden's 1772 account of chest pain occurring in "nearly a hundred people"[2]:

> There is a disorder of the breast marked with strong and peculiar symptoms, considerable for the kind of danger belonging to it, and not extremely rare....They who are afflicted with it, are seized while they are walking (more especially if it be up hill, and soon after eating) with a painful and most disagreeable sensation in the breast which seems as if it would extinguish life, if it were to increase or to continue; but the moment they stand still, all this uneasiness vanishes....In some inveterate cases it has been brought on by the motion of a horse, or a carriage, and even by swallowing, coughing, going to stool, or speaking, or any disturbance of mind.

This elegant description turns out to be the first delineation of the syndrome of angina pectoris.

More recently, a group of New York physicians noticed an unusual cluster of patients with a rare skin tumor.[3] Not only was the frequency of these cases unexpected, but the course of the disease was atypical. Where the malignancy usually occurs as a slowly growing affliction of men in their sixties or seventies, it suddenly presented as an aggressive, life-threatening disease among homosexual men in their twenties and thirties. Needless to say, this description of eight cases of Kaposi's sarcoma first alerted the world to a problem of considerable importance.

Another type of descriptive study is the clinical series in which a physician describes the outcome of 100 patients undergoing a new technique for snaring gallstones or how 50 snakebite victims were treated—not fancy research, but useful catalogs of the experience of others. Some merits of these later.

Large populations can also be the subject of descriptive studies. Collecting diagnostic information on a practice population by counting the number of hypertensives, diabetics, and patients with acute sore throat seen over a period of time has been used for "defining the content of family practice."[4] This type of information helps in making practice-management decisions, such as the need for a dietitian to counsel diabetics or how to plan a curriculum for training residents. A description of a new course in human sexuality that has been successfully taught to medical students or a community survey conducted to assess the health needs of the geriatric population are other examples of this type of design. So, in addition to being starting points for more elaborate assaults on the etiology of disease, descriptive studies can be used for a variety of educational, administrative, and health-planning purposes.

EXPLANATORY STUDIES

Comparison is the basic strategy of explanatory studies. Such studies seek answers to such questions as: Which treatment for breast cancer is most effective? Is there a relationship between use of oral hypoglycemics and heart disease? What are the factors that predict which patients will miss appointments? Explanatory studies attempt to provide insight into etiology or find better treatments. The methods employed can be grouped into two major approaches, as seen on the right-hand side of Table 2-1.

Experimental studies

The first of the explanatory study designs is the experimental strategy, which is familiar to most of us from undergraduate chemistry or psychology. In medical research it travels under the aliases of the controlled trial, clinical trial, health-care trial, or intervention trial. The primary feature that distinguishes the controlled trial from other explanatory studies is the active intervention of the investigator. The researcher gives an antidepressant medication to one group of volunteers and a placebo to another group; one-half of a medical-school class is selected to receive a new self-instructional package on anemia while the other half gets a lecture; patients in a practice are randomly assigned to a physician or to a nurse practitioner for care. In each case, the researcher who is testing the efficacy of the method is able to exercise control by assigning subjects to medications, lectures, or nurse practitioners. Figure 2-1 illustrates the general outline of the con-

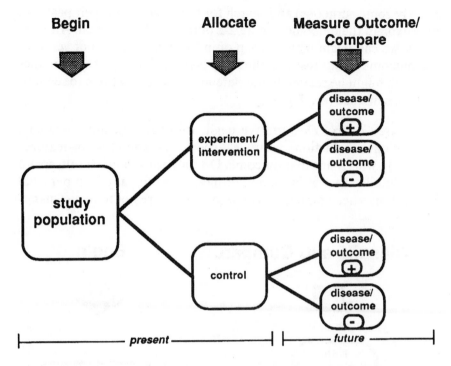

Begin　　　　**Allocate**　　　**Measure Outcome/ Compare**

FIGURE 2-1 **Experimental or controlled trial design.**

trolled trial. It is an extremely important form of study design and will be dealt with in more detail later.

Observational studies

Observational studies also utilize comparisons to examine and explain medical mysteries. However, unlike the controlled trial, the observational study relegates researchers to the role of bystanders. They study the natural course of health events, gather data about subjects, and classify and sort them. By the strategy of making comparisons, they then try to provide insights into the cause of diseases.

The plethora of terms at the beginning of this chapter notwithstanding, there are really only two fundamental ways of approaching an observational study. We can start by studying individuals who already have a particular disease or outcome (patients with toxemia of pregnancy or low satisfaction with medical care, or doctors who have become surgeons) and search for some factors in their past that may explain the outcome. Figure 2-2 outlines this approach. Alternatively, we can begin with a group of individuals who do not yet have the outcome of interest, examine and classify them by characteristics we think might be related to the outcome, and follow them to see who develops disease (see Fig. 2-3).

The Case-Control Design We begin with the outcome—toxemia, low patient satisfaction, or surgical specialty—and look for features of people who share that outcome. Do they eat too much salt, spend more time in the waiting room, or have exceptionally high personal motivation when compared with people who are not toxemic, dissat-

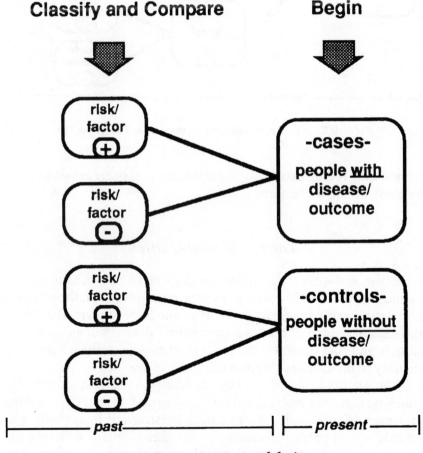

FIGURE 2-2 Case-control design.

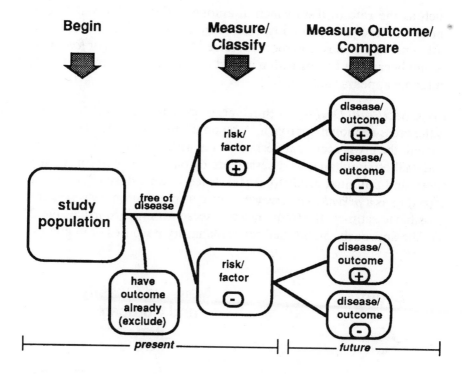

FIGURE 2-3 Follow-up design.

isfied, or surgeons? If differences in frequencies of the characteristics between the cases and the comparison group are found, we have taken a positive step toward explaining the outcome. We will call this the *case-control approach*, although it should be clear from the examples used that the term *case* is used broadly to define an individual who already has the outcome of interest. That outcome need not be a medical disease. The term *case-control* does convey the major activity of the design: that we begin at the end with people who have the outcome and compare their characteristics with subjects who do not (see Fig. 2-2).

Follow-up Design We begin with people who have not yet experienced the outcome: patients early in pregnancy, new registrants in a practice, or third-year medical students. Characteristics of the group, such as diet, waiting time, or motivation, are measured and cataloged, and the researcher sits back and watches for toxemia, dissatisfaction, or choice of medical specialty to develop. Again, using comparisons, such as the rate of dissatisfaction among patients who wait against those who are seen promptly, light is shed on possible causes of the outcome. This is most commonly referred to as the *cohort* or *follow-up design* because it begins with a cohort or group and follows it till the outcome appears (see Fig. 2-3).

Cross-Sectional Design A third variation on the observational study is the cross-sectional approach. A blend of the two strategies just discussed, the cross-sectional design begins with a population or cohort and makes simultaneous assessments of outcomes, descriptive features, and potential predictors. This "slice-in-time design" is also referred to as a *prevalence survey*, because its population basis makes it possible to estimate the frequency of disease within a group (see Fig. 2-4). The approach can be used for explanatory purposes or in giving a

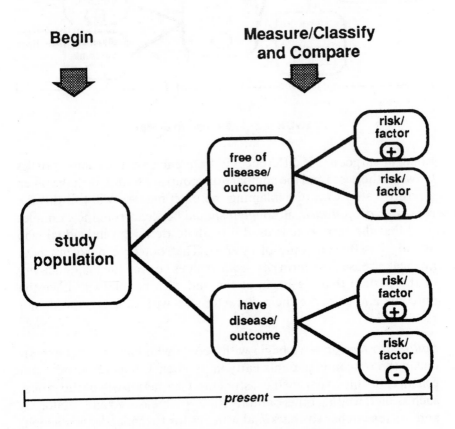

FIGURE 2-4 Cross-sectional design.

descriptive account of an outcome or disease. A community survey of blood lead levels in young children identifies the extent (prevalence) of lead poisoning in the community and assesses the need for medical services. If information is obtained on the children's environment, the cause of elevated blood lead levels can also be evaluated.

A Concocted Example

For purposes of illustration, we can take a single example and try out each of the major explanatory approaches. To give us a working terminology, we will call them experimental, case-control, and follow-up designs.

The Problem   During the past few years of practice, we have made a fascinating clinical observation. In talking to patients who suffer from poor visual acuity and wear glasses, we have noted that their diets seem to be remarkably deficient in carrots. Now everyone knows that the carotenes that give carrots their lovely orange glow are essential for the formation of rhodopsin, a retinal pigment associated with good night vision, but it appears we are onto the illuminating discovery that previously unappreciated components of carrots may actually aid visual acuity. In fact, our first informal survey revealed that of five bespectacled patients queried, all admitted to a singular disinterest in carrots. The question is how to pursue this exciting hunch and create an explanatory study that will substantiate our hypothesis that an association exists between good vision and carrot consumption.

Case-control design   We begin by collecting 100 of our spectacle-wearing patients to represent the cases. They already have the outcome—poor visual acuity. As a comparison or control group, we identify another 100 individuals—patients who are generally like our first group except that they enjoy 20/20 vision. We then proceed to ask each of these 200 people to give us an exhaustive accounting of their dietary habits over recent years, paying particular attention to their consumption of carrots. Our hope will be that a conspicuous difference in carrot eating will be found between those with good and those with poor vision. If the patients with poor vision are well below the comparison group with respect to carrot intake, we will have evidence to support the link between carrots and eyesight. Figure 2-5 reflects all this.

Follow-up design Figure 2-6 shows how our example might look as a follow-up study. All patients who enter the practice will be given a test for visual acuity. Subjects who already have poor acuity will be dropped from further consideration. They already have the outcome. For the remainder, those with good vision, dietary records will be maintained so we will have an accurate account of the carrot intake of all our subjects. These people will be followed for the next 10 years, and at the end of that time everyone's vision will be retested. Armed

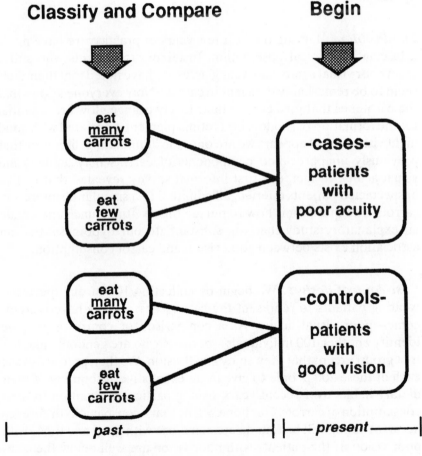

FIGURE 2-5 Case-control design.

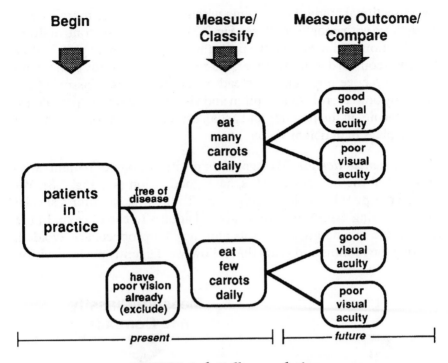

FIGURE 2-6 Follow-up design.

with information on carrot consumption with which to classify subjects, we will be able to compare the vision status of patients with high intake with that of patients who eat few or no carrots at all. If carrot eaters see better than those who eschew the orange roots, our hypothesis will be supported. It should be emphasized that the follow-up design just described is an observational rather than experimental study, despite the fact that as investigators we seemed to be assuming a very active role. We examined eyesight and counted carrots, but we never told our patients how many carrots they should eat. That was left to nature.

Cross-sectional design   On the way to performing our follow-up study we dismissed the portion of our population who were screened and found lacking in visual acuity. We could have gained some information from this group, however. Had we taken the trouble to ask them about their current carrot-eating habits, we could have compared their intake with the carrot consumption of patients with good eyesight. This slice of information from our practice would be a cross-sectional study: Do patients with good vision eat more carrots than those with poor vision? (see Fig. 2-7). As in the case-control study, information on diet is from the past, albeit the immediate past. Unlike the case-control design, however, the cross-sectional study begins with a large practice population instead of selected cases. Classifying patients by both carrot consumption and vision, we learn the prevalence of low acuity in the practice and get an estimate of the role that carrot eating plays in deficient vision.

Experimental design We again begin with a group of patients who are free of the outcome, that is, have good vision (see Fig. 2-8). We divide our population into two groups. To the first we offer a special diet including everything from carrot daiquiris to carrot cake. In the diet of the second group, carrots and their by-products are avoided. During the months and years that follow, we diligently perform vision

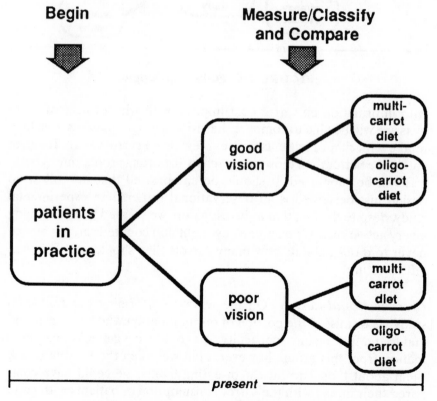

FIGURE 2-7 Cross-sectional design.

Begin

Allocate

**Measure Outcome/
Compare**

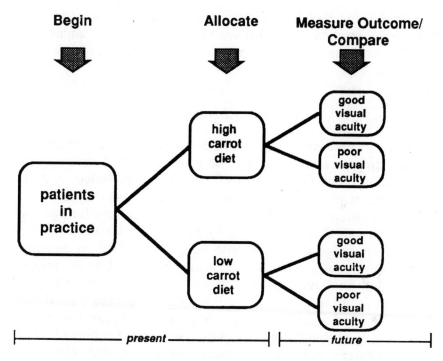

FIGURE 2-8 Experimental or controlled trial design.

examinations to see how our two groups fare and ultimately compare the high- and low-carrot-diet groups with respect to vision outcomes.

Each of these strategies has a distinctive flavor. The case-control format has an economy about it, but one can sense difficulties in retrieving information from the past and in finding proper groups to compare. The follow-up and experimental designs allow better planning and control but require ongoing diligence to keep track of subjects and see that people stay on their diets. We will examine the advantages of the different methodologies as well as explore their limitations and tribulations in the next few chapters.

MORE CONFUSING TERMINOLOGY

Identifying study designs can be a perplexing business. Even people who ought to know better occasionally get caught with their terms in a tangle. Bits of jargon that are particularly troublesome are the duos: Cases and controls, and prospective and retrospective. The ambiguous use of these terms accounts for much confusion, pain, and suffering.

Cases and controls

Take, for example, an article that gives itself simultaneous billing as a "long-term case-control study" and an account of the "natural history of bacteriuria in schoolgirls."[5] Now pause and reflect. A study tracking the natural history of something sounds like it ought to be following a group of subjects with a certain characteristic for a period of time to see what happens to them. It does not sound like a case-control design that starts with people who have an outcome and tries to discover past habits that may be related. Sure enough, in this study the investigators evaluated a group of 60 schoolgirls who were found through a screening program to have bacteriuria, then reexamined them periodically for a number of years to see who developed renal complications. Complication rates for girls who had bacteriuria were found to be substantially higher when compared with rates for a group of girls who were without infections. A perfect example of a follow-up study!

The confusion arises because of the use of the term "case" to describe girls who have bacteriuria. They are indeed cases as the clinician uses the term to identify patients who have a disease or health condition. They are not cases, however, in the sense the researcher uses the term to define a group with an outcome that will serve as a starting point for a comparative study. Bacteriuria is not the outcome of this observational study. The outcome is chronic renal disease. Bacteriuria is a characteristic shared by a portion of the initial cohort of schoolgirls that we wish to follow. At the same time, controls as used in this paper are really a subset of girls from a larger population who were screened for urinary-tract infection and found free of bacteriuria. They are followed forward in time for comparative purposes and assessed for renal complications. They are not the foils in a case-control design.

To quibble with Gertrude Stein a bit—a case is not a case is not a case. Sometimes a case is a subject in a specific explanatory strategy who has been chosen because she has the outcome under study—toxemia, low satisfaction, or poor visual acuity. Sometimes that same toxemia, low satisfaction, or poor visual acuity is the starting point of the study and groups of cases that share a characteristic are watched for development of outcomes, such as perinatal death, broken appointments, or traffic accidents. Readers must avoid the temptation to classify every article that refers to cases and controls as a case-control study. It may be a follow-up or experimental design.

Prospective and retrospective

Perhaps the most confusing of all terminology encountered in descriptions of medical studies are references to prospective and retrospective designs. It does not take an etymologist to tell you that these two words describe a relationship to time—looking forward in time and looking backward. Unfortunately, in common medical usage they have also come to be synonyms for design structures. Studies we call case-control designs are also known as retrospective studies; those that we designate as cohort or follow-up studies are also referred to as prospective studies.

Time can be a bugbear unless readers keep the time frame in which a study is conducted separate from the strategy of comparison that is being used. Retrospective studies begin and end in the present but involve a major backward glance to collect information about events that occurred in the past. Prospective studies also begin in the present but march forward, collecting data about a population whose outcome lies in the future. But these two terms do not offer sufficient precision about the strategy of the study. It should be clear, for example, that both the controlled trial and the follow-up design proceed in a prospective, forward fashion. Both these strategies begin with a population, gather measurements, and watch for developments in the future, but conceptually experimental versus observational strategies are different.

Similarly, the notion that any study that uses data which are collected retrospectively falls into the case-control category is misleading. One design that is becoming increasingly popular utilizes the follow-up technique but does it using information from the past. This strategy labors under the awkward designation of retrospective follow-up, historical prospective, or retrospective cohort design. The key to the success of this approach (as diagrammed in Fig. 2-9) is the availability of carefully kept records from the past.

Begin　　　　**Measure/**　　**Measure Outcome/**
　　　　　　　　　Classify　　　　**Compare**

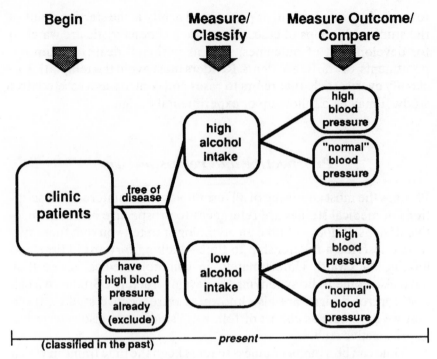

FIGURE 2-9 Restrospective follow-up design.

Researchers wishing to examine the relationship between alcohol consumption and development of high blood pressure might need to wait 20 years before patients they have screened and classified with respect to alcohol consumption develop high blood pressure. If, however, they can find medical records that document the drinking habits and blood pressures of people 15 to 20 years ago, they can greatly condense the time frame of the study. They select a cohort of people whose alcohol consumption was conscientiously recorded in 1960, follow them up to the present by measuring current blood pressures, and produce a retrospective follow-up study.

A number of authors[6-11] have written in some detail about the confusion resulting from mixing connotations of time with references to design strategy. It is best for purposes of clarity to reduce prospective and retrospective to their roles as clock watchers and employ other terms to describe study plans.

Table 2-2 attempts to place the terminology chaos in some order. In it, designs have been grouped into categories that should be most

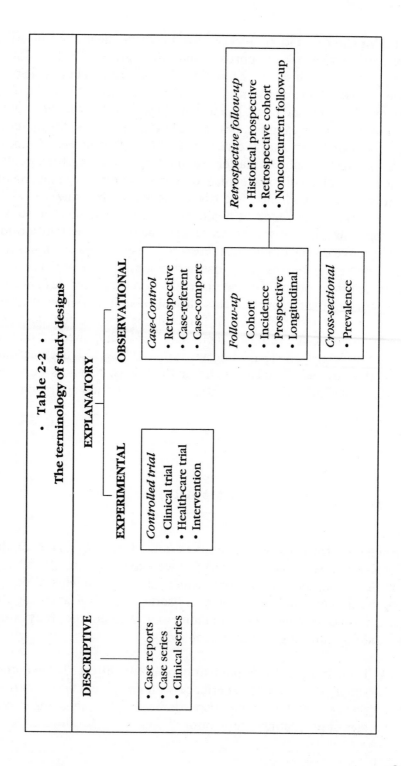

• Table 2-2 •
The terminology of study designs

DESCRIPTIVE

- Case reports
- Case series
- Clinical series

EXPLANATORY

EXPERIMENTAL

Controlled trial
- Clinical trial
- Health-care trial
- Intervention

OBSERVATIONAL

Case-Control
- Retrospective
- Case-referent
- Case-compere

Follow-up
- Cohort
- Incidence
- Prospective
- Longitudinal

Cross-sectional
- Prevalence

Retrospective follow-up
- Historical prospective
- Retrospective cohort
- Nonconcurrent follow-up

useful for clinical readers. Terms we will be using head the lists, with synonyms or relatives in approach and intent grouped below. Some may object to such insensitive lumping of so large a number of elegant terms. Indeed, there are some fine distinctions within the groupings that have been passed over. The terminology used to describe experimental studies, for example, has expanded to encompass the increasing variety of topics that the design has come to address. "Clinical trials" suggests a subject matter confined to evaluating therapeutic maneuvers with traditional clinical outcomes, like relief of angina or improved survival. Health-care trials, it is argued by Spitzer et al.,[12] evaluate a broader range of health outcomes, including "personal, sociologic, administrative, and economic data that are seldom considered in conventional biomedical research." They cite as examples the trials comparing the use of nurse practitioners with physicians in medical settings or trials of patient-education programs designed to improve compliance. Experiments have also been undertaken to test the value of geriatric assessment teams, home visits to families with newborn babies, and differing methods of providing medical education to physicians. The term "intervention trial" has also been used to imply the broadened scope of the methodology. Nuances notwithstanding, all share a common controlled, experimental approach.

SUMMARY

Having gone through the strenuous exercise of pinning a label on the structure of a study, what reward can we expect for the effort? The next three chapters will burrow deeper into the problems of design and, it is hoped, will come out with useful advice for assessing the strengths and weaknesses of common designs. To put the study into a methodological category ask the following:

1. Is the design a descriptive or explanatory effort? Is the author simply detailing an experience with cases, practices, or treatments or making comparisons in hopes of establishing etiologies or evaluating interventions?

2. If comparisons are being made, is the investigator observing the course of events or creating an experiment by assigning subjects to receive a pill, an exercise program, or a piece of health advice?

3. If the design is observational, are patients who already have a disease or outcome compared with unaffected controls for preexisting characteristics? Or do investigators classify and follow a cohort of subjects for development of the outcome or effect of interest?

REFERENCES

1. Lilienfeld DE: Definitions of epidemiology. *Am J Epidemiol* 107:87, 1978.
2. Heberden W: Commentaries on the history and cure of diseases, in Willius FA, Keys TE(eds): *Classics of Cardiology*, vol. 1. New York, Dover Publications, 1961.
3. Hymes KB, Greene JB, Marcus A, et al: Kaposi's sarcoma in homosexual men—A report of eight cases. *Lancet* 2:598, 1981.
4. Marsland DW, Wood M, Mayo F: Content of family practice. *J Fam Pract* 3:37, 1976.
5. Gillenwater JY, Harrison RB, Kunin CM: Natural history of bacteriuria in schoolgirls. A long-term case-control study. *N Engl J Med* 301:396, 1979.
6. Clark VA, Hopkins CE: Time is of the essence. *J Chron Dis* 20:565, 1967.
7. Feinstein AR: Directionality and scientific inference. *J Clin Epidemiol* 42:829, 1989.
8. Greenland S, Morgenstern H: What is directionality? *J Clin Epidemiol* 42:821, 1989.
9. Kramer MS, Boivin J: Directionality, timing, and sample selection in epidemiologic research design. *J Clin Epidemiol* 42:827, 1989.
10. Kramer MS, Boivin J: Toward an "unconfounded" classification of epidemiologic research design. *J Chron Dis* 40:683, 1987.
11. Sartwell PE: Retrospective studies: A review for the clinician. *Ann Intern Med* 81:381, 1974.
12. Spitzer WO, Feinstein AR, Sackett DL: What is a health care trial? *JAMA* 233:161, 1975.

CHAPTER THREE

STUDY DESIGN: THE CASE-CONTROL APPROACH

... you yourself sir, should be as old as I am if, like a crab, you could go backward.

HAMLET, Act II, Scene II

Case-control studies have been much maligned. Who among us has not experienced the dismay of making a particularly bright remark referencing Dr. Rasputin's work on hemophilia, only to hear ourselves rebuffed by the ultimate put-down, "Of course those were retrospective studies." The implication is clear. Nothing could be a cruder masquerade for a research study than a retrospective or case-control effort. It is surprising how common this notion is. Some people continue to argue that satisfactory solutions to research questions can never be obtained through the case-control methodology because there are insurmountable problems in going backward.

It is well to clear our heads now of sweeping prejudices against the case-control design. For although the method falls prey to a number of difficulties, it has become standard fare. Cole reports a four- to seven-fold increase in the number of case-control reports published in *Lancet* over the 20-year period 1956–1976.[1] During this same time, the *American Journal of Epidemiology* also showed an increase in the use of the design among its published articles. With the rising costs of performing long-term, follow-up studies on large populations, the case-control design will probably find even greater use in the future. The method has some very compelling features that should be recognized before we start going after the tender points.

ADVANTAGES OF THE CASE-CONTROL DESIGN

The case-control design is ideally suited for initial, explanatory ventures. As we have seen with Hymes's observations on Kaposi's sarcoma[2] or the example of carrots and vision, many important medical discoveries begin with a clinical observation or hunch. An unusual clustering of cases of cancer is noted, a surprising side effect is observed following the use of an antibiotic, a group of children with learning disabilities are reported to have been formula fed as infants. The handiest way to see if these hunches lead to valid discoveries is to make some quick comparisons with subjects who are readily at hand. Are patients with mesothelioma more likely to have been exposed to asbestos than a comparison group? Is there a difference in the history of breast and bottle feeding between children with learning disabilities and those who perform well in school? The case-control design is ideal for trying these hypotheses. It is very *efficient*. Since our novel observations generally begin with patients who have experienced the unusual disease or side effect, collecting cases is relatively easy. Hospitals and out-patient clinics are replete with patients who already have diseases or outcomes we may wish to study. We need not wait years for the outcome to develop or expend great energy tracking down subjects who require follow-up.

Another widely advertised advantage of the case-control design is its *utility for studying rare diseases*. This point certainly appears to have merit, since even the most common diseases occur relatively infrequently. The annual incidence of breast cancer, for example, is about 85 per 100,000 women; only about 1 in 100 men between 50 and 59 years of age will have a heart attack each year. This means that, to perform follow-up studies, extremely large populations must be monitored to supply even a small handful of cases.

The case-control approach is also conducive to voyages into the uncharted waters of disease etiology. To this end, in anticipation of future explorations, large data banks have been collected detailing all sorts of information on patients from their habits of alcohol consumption to their zoonotic afflictions. Rather than beginning with a hunch they wish to test, investigators engage in "hypothesis generation" or what some disparage as "data dredging" or "fishing."[3] Patients with a disease such as endometrial cancer are culled from the data base and a list of their behavioral and pharmacological exposures is compared to the exposure frequencies of a control group selected from the same data base. Many comparisons are made, and sometimes, by virtue of persistence and force of numbers, associations between a medication or habit and the disease are discovered.

PROBLEMS OF CASE-CONTROL DESIGNS

The objective of the case-control design is to identify causes of a disease or other outcome. The strategy is to compare the frequency of a risk factor among those who are afflicted compared with those who are not. All other things being equal (which is not always the case), differential rates of exposure point to etiology. If dissatisfied patients wait twice as long in the waiting room as those who are pleased with their care, or women with toxemia eat half again as much salt as women who have uneventful pregnancies, we have evidence that increased waiting time and high-salt diets may be responsible for the adverse outcomes. Critiques of the case-control methodology have been written, which include thought-provoking discussions of both basics and subtleties.[1,4] Essential to the validity of case-control designs is the appropriate selection of cases and controls, and the adequacy and comparability of the exposure data obtained. We will look at these issues in turn.

Selection of cases

Sample selection The choice of cases can create difficulties if those sampled do not represent the larger population of those who have the outcome. A highly screened sample, such as patients admitted to a referral hospital, may not offer an accurate reflection of the world of patients with rheumatoid arthritis or type I diabetes.

A case-control study that was designed to discover whether maternal smoking and alcohol consumption during pregnancy predisposes infants to febrile seizures illustrates this problem.[5] Febrile seizure cases in this endeavor were identified primarily through emergency room log books from 20 western Washington hospitals. For each childhood seizure case, a control was recruited, using birth records of infants born at the same hospital during the same week. When control candidates could not be contacted or declined participation, investigators returned to the birth registries and identified another child born as proximate to the case as possible. Telephone interviews were conducted with mothers of both groups. Prenatal histories of health habits, including use of alcohol and tobacco during pregnancy, were obtained. Results indicated that mothers of seizure infants were more likely to have smoked cigarettes and consumed alcohol during pregnancy than comparison mothers. Babies born to these women were twice as likely as comparison infants to experience febrile seizures—further evidence for the adverse consequences of smoking and drinking during pregnancy. However, a critical commentary published with this report[6] suggests that bias may have crept in when cases were chosen. The critique points out that many children with febrile seizures are not seen in emergency rooms. Those who do seek emergency room care are often from families without regular physicians, families who may be less health-conscious in other health behaviors, such as smoking and drinking. This would mean that estimates of alcohol and tobacco use from this sample of mothers would be spuriously high. The subsequent calculation of excess risk would be exaggerated.

It is also important that cases not be identified *because* of their exposure. If the knowledge that a subject has a potential risk factor *prompts* diagnosis of the disease or outcome, study validity may be jeopardized. The editors of the *Journal of the American Medical Association* provided an illustration when they published two papers with differing views on the role of tampons in the etiology of toxic shock syndrome (TSS). The first paper came from the Centers for Disease Control (CDC)[7] and was one of several case-control studies that looked for risk factors for TSS. Using the classic case-control approach, investigators identified patients whose episodes of TSS had been reported to the CDC. The 50 women selected were asked to identify 3 acquaintances of approximately the same age who lived in the same geographic area. These friends formed a control group. Cases and controls were interviewed by telephone and asked to identify the type of "menstrual device" used during the month in which the woman became ill. All 50 of the selected cases but only 125 of 150 controls had used tampons during their menstrual period. This finding created a significant association between tampon use and the development of TSS.

In the same issue of the journal, a group from Yale University critically reviewed publications that linked toxic shock and tampon use,[8] noting that bias might have occurred because of the way cases were identified. Early reports linking the syndrome to menstruation and possibly to tampon use had received wide publicity by the time several of the research studies had begun. A *diagnostic bias* might have occurred if patients with equivocal criteria for TSS were given the diagnosis *because* they were known to be menstruating and using tampons. The critics cited an example where a woman whose symptoms were, in fact, most suggestive of *Shigella* enteritis was diagnosed as TSS for just such reasons. *Reporting bias* might also be present and work in a similar fashion. Because of the publicity implicating menstruation and tampon use as risks for TSS, physicians might have been more likely to report an episode to CDC if the patient's history was positive for these two features.

Case definitions Cases need to be carefully defined. Is the author talking about a clearly delineated, homogeneous problem? Is a single outcome being considered, or are multiple, related conditions, which might have different etiologies, being inappropriately lumped together? No one would consider a case-control study that combined cases of leukemia, Wilms's tumor, and colorectal cancer in a single category. Even with a specific tumor site, we know that etiology may differ depending upon the histologic type. Asking patients with adenocarcinoma of the lung about their past cigarette smoking may yield one result, and the same question posed to a group of patients with squamous cell lung cancer may yield quite another. The strong association between smoking and lung cancer holds primarily for the latter tumor.

If the sample of cases is diluted by the unwitting inclusion of subjects who do not truly have the disease or outcome of interest, a true association between the exposure and disease may be missed. In the large U.S. Public Health Service study that explored the relationship between Reye's syndrome and medication use,[9] 70 pediatric referral centers were enlisted to identify this unusual but life-threatening childhood illness. Because the disease—which is characterized by a sudden, unexpected deterioration in mental status following a mild respiratory or gastrointestinal illness—might be confused with other conditions, investigators were careful to include as cases only subjects who met rigorous criteria and passed review of a physician panel. As it happened, 53 patients were reported through the hospital network, but only 27 met the standards as bona fide cases of Reye's and were included in the final study. It is easy to imagine that the medication histories of the 26 excluded might have been dissimilar. So although it appears that something was lost by reducing the number of study cases, the increased confidence that a homogeneous disease entity was being evaluated more than compensated. Had the other 26 reported "cases" been included, overall exposure frequencies to aspirin would likely have been less than the 96 percent that was found and the strong association would have been substantially reduced.

Selection of controls

The choice of an appropriate control group is also a challenging proposition. The idea, of course, is to find a group of individuals who come from the same general population as cases but who do not have heart disease, bronchitis, or low satisfaction. Our need is to derive an estimate of "general" rates of exposure to high-fat diets, secondhand smoke, or prolonged waiting room time. Finding a group that represents this "general population" is more difficult than one might think. The choice of controls can bias results by selectively including subjects who either underestimate or overestimate exposures.

One commonly utilized source of control subjects which is notorious for creating this dilemma is the hospital. Because patients with serious diseases are easy to locate in hospitals, selecting controls from the same hospital population is not only convenient but sensible. Subjects in the same facility are likely to come from the same community and have similar access to the health system. When investigators from Boston explored the relationship between coffee consumption and cancer of the pancreas, they found histories of higher coffee intake among cancer patients than among controls.[10] Cases of pancreatic cancer were obtained from 11 large metropolitan hospitals. Controls were selected from patients who were under the care of the same physician in the same hospital as cases. It turned out that "because of the nature of practices of many of the physicians..., patients with gastroenterologic conditions were probably overrepresented in relation to a general hospital population."[10] These included patients with hernia, colitis, enteritis, diverticulitis, and a variety of other conditions. The authors themselves expressed concern that the coffee-drinking habits of such a control group might not represent those of the population at large. Patients with gastroenterologic problems may not drink much coffee, either because it worsens their condition or because their doctors admonished them against coffee use. If coffee intake by controls is spuriously low, that of cancer patients appears elevated in comparison, and a false association between coffee and pancreatic cancer results.

Silverman et al.[11] studied the prevalence of coffee drinking among hospitalized and population-based groups. Using data from a national study conducted in the Detroit area, they found that the pattern of coffee drinking among all hospitalized patients was similar to that in the overall population. However, in the subgroup of patients with digestive disorders, the number of cups of coffee taken per day was significantly lower. Only 55 percent of hospitalized patients with gastrointestinal problems drank two or more cups of coffee per day compared with 73 percent of population controls. The difference in coffee-drinking habits of patients with pancreatic cancer and controls may thus not be due to a link between the beverage and the disease but rather to the selection of a control group with an unusually low prevalence of the risk factor.*

An inappropriate control group can have the opposite effect and obscure an important link between a disease and its cause. Suppose, for example, that hospitalized lung cancer patients were questioned regarding their smoking habits. If the reports of these patients were compared with those of hospital patients who did not have cancer, the connection between smoking and lung cancer might appear to be spuriously low. Many hospitalized patients may be suffering from other smoking-related diseases, such as emphysema, bronchitis, or heart disease. They may admit to cigarette usage every bit as high as that of patients with lung cancer, and the strong association between smoking and cancer that would appear if a population of healthy controls were used is lost.

---

*The coffee/pancreatic cancer story is continued in Chap. 13.

Alleviating control-group problems

Multiple controls   One approach to warding off the demons of control selection is to employ more than one control group. *Multiple control groups* can offer independent estimates of exposure among different samples of noncases and substantially strengthen a study's findings. The Public Health Service study of Reye's syndrome and medications is a creative illustration.[9] Rather than settle for a single control group, researchers enlisted subjects to represent four different populations. All controls were children of approximately the same age as case subjects. All had recently had a respiratory or gastrointestinal illness. But because investigators were concerned about the selective forces that place some children with respiratory illness in hospitals while others remain at home and the relevance that this might have to medication use, they chose a spectrum of control subjects.

Children who are patients in referral centers are likely to have illnesses that are comparable in severity to Reye's syndrome and so make logical controls. But this group may overrepresent children with chronic illnesses who may be on *more* medications than a typical child or may have been instructed to *avoid* certain drugs. Emergency room patients constituted another group. Such sick children are easy to locate, have antecedent illnesses that are more like those of the cases in severity, but have a lower burden of chronic disease. Two other groups were obtained to offer a picture of more general medication use, one from among children attending the same school or day care center as the case and the other from a random-digit-dialing telephone survey. These children were clearly much less severely ill than Reye's cases. With four control groups, four estimates of "general" medication use were available.

Results were dramatic. Ninety-six percent of Reye's syndrome patients reported use of salicylates, compared with only 40 percent of emergency room controls and 44 and 35 percent of school and random-digit-dialing telephone controls, respectively. Only 27 percent of hospital controls had been given salicylates. The relatively consistent rate of control-group exposure using these very different populations strengthens one's confidence that the exposures of the two groups were truly different. Rates of medications other than salicylates were also tallied and found to be *similar* across case and control groups. An exception was acetaminophen, an analgesic/antipyretic substitute for aspirin, where usage was considerably *higher* for controls than cases (see Table 3-1). All this serves to further enhance the association between salicylate use and Reye's.

Community controls The use of *community controls* has been one approach to attempting to find more accurate estimates of exposure among the non-ill for comparison purposes. Community controls are frequently obtained from the neighborhoods or social groups from which cases come. They can also be recruited through random community surveys conducted by mail or telephone.

In a paper that attempted to determine environmental and social features that distinguished children seen in a psychiatric outpatient clinic from other children,[12] a sample of children seen in several psychiatric outpatient facilities was contrasted with two control groups. The first was a hospital control group that consisted of children from the pediatric clinic, children from the ophthalmology clinic, and children who had had an appendectomy or tonsillectomy. The second group came from the same neighborhood as the cases but was not part of an identified hospital or clinic population. The authors queried parents of the children in each of these three groups about a host of factors, ranging from whether the child had nightmares and temper tantrums to the marital relationship of the parents, the child's progress in school, and whether or not the child was spanked. Not surprisingly,

---

• **TABLE 3-1** •

Medication exposures of Reye's syndrome cases and four control groups

Medication	Cases ($n=27$)	Controls[a]				
		Inpatient ($n=22$)	ER ($n=30$)	School ($n=45$)	Community ($n=43$)	Total ($n=140$)
Acetaminophen	26.9	77.3	90.0	91.1	81.4	85.7
Chlorpheniramine	22.2	22.7	23.3	20.0	37.2	26.4
Phenylephrine	14.8	22.7	6.7	20.0	20.9	17.9
Pseudoephedrine	29.6	31.8	16.7	26.7	48.8	32.1
Salicylates/aspirin	96.3	27.3	40.0	44.4	34.9	37.9

[a]Controls obtained from hospital inpatient and emergency rooms (ER), schools, and random-digit-dialing telephone survey (Community).

Source: Adapted from Hurwitz et al.[9]

children from the psychiatric clinic showed more problem behaviors and disrupted families than control children. However, a "striking and unexpected finding was the difference between the hospital control and community control [patients]." Factors such as parental loss, fears, temper tantrums, nightmares, and reports of maladjustment by teachers occurred much more frequently among control children chosen from the clinics than among those taken from the neighborhood. The difference was seen despite the intentional selection of hospital controls who had minor illnesses and surgical procedures. It suggests that children who get into the medical system, regardless of the reason, have characteristics that differ from those of a group of community kids.

The hazard in using community controls lies not in the source but in the sampling. It is critical that community subjects who are located through surveys and who agree to participate in the study present a representative risk profile. Individuals without telephones cannot be included in a random-digit-dialing survey. Employed people may not be at home if contact is attempted during working hours. Some may simply find participation too onerous, too threatening, or too unimportant. If these folks have different habits, beliefs, and behaviors from individuals who are successfully contacted and agree to serve as control subjects, the community is not being reflected accurately.

The study linking maternal alcohol and tobacco use to febrile seizures was criticized for its selection of controls as well as cases.[6] Researchers attempted to enlist controls through telephone and mail contact. If a potential control could not be reached or refused participation, another possible subject was chosen and enrollment attempts repeated until the full complement of control subjects was obtained. Over 1050 potential controls were screened in order to enroll 472 subjects. It is argued[6] that the low enrollment rate opens the way for bias. Individuals who agreed to participate as control subjects are likely to be more health-conscious than those who could not be located or refused participation. Smoking and alcohol consumption could well be underrepresented among this group and could increase the exposure contrast between cases and controls.

Matching One way of dealing with factors that may confuse the comparison between cases and controls is to employ a technique known as *matching*. This is a term frequently encountered in descriptions of study methods. It means that investigators have made an effort to select control subjects who share particular characteristics with the cases. Matching has a specific purpose. It improves the efficiency of a study by keeping constant or controlling factors that are known to be related to the outcome and may confound or confuse results if they occur disproportionately in the groups that are being compared.

Suppose we wish to evaluate a hunch we have developed that cigar smoking causes people to lose their hair. To study this question in the case-control mode, we first select a group of balding patients from the dermatology clinic—patients who are undergoing a fancy hair-implantation procedure. As soon as they feel up to wrinkling their brows, we quiz them about their past habits, making special note of cigar smoking. We then need to ask the same questions of a comparison group. A little thought suggests that trotting down the hallway to the pediatric clinic would be unwise. The youngsters there, although clinic patients, bear little resemblance to the patients undergoing hair transplants. The obvious difference, age, is an important one because it is related to the habit and the outcome. Cigar smoking is an activity that increases with age; so does baldness. One would expect a higher rate of cigar smoking among the dermatology clinic patients because they are older, not because cigars cause baldness. We would be ill advised to advertise a link between stogie puffing and alopecia without some way of accounting for the role of age.

Matching reduces competing explanations for the outcome in question. If we selected age-matched controls to compare with our bald patients—that is, if we chose subjects who were close in age to our cases—we would eliminate or control any confusion about whether it is really smoking or just age that is related to hair loss. If we still found higher smoking rates among cases, it would not be because of differential ages in the groups. This kind of matching may be done on a case-by-case basis, where each bald patient is matched with a hairy subject who is within one or two years of being the same age. It may also be accomplished in groups, where both cases and controls are chosen from patients who fall within a specified age range. Age is probably the most commonly matched variable because it is related to so many habits and diseases that come under study. Sex, race, and socioeconomic status are other commonly used variables, but matching may be carried out on any factor, from apple-cider drinking to exposure to zinc smelters. It is a lovely technique for creating order in the world. However, there is a price to be paid for matching.

Overmatching An investigator can overmatch. Matching equalizes the occurrence of a factor in the groups that are being compared; therefore, once cases and controls are matched by age, sex, or whatever, these factors can no longer be evaluated as possible etiologic agents. As an obvious example, suppose we are fledgling hematologists, unencumbered by previous knowledge about causes of anemia. We have discovered a group of patients with severe anemia who have unusual, sickle-shaped red cells in their blood smears. In an attempt to learn more about the etiology of this disease, we devise a clever case-control, observational study in which we match patients who have the anemia with nonanemic medical patients of the same age, race, and sex. We note in passing that the cases all happen to be black and, therefore, we select only blacks as control patients. We have overmatched. By matching for race we have lost our ability to show that sickle-cell anemia has a genetic basis as reflected by differential occurrence in whites and blacks.

Ascertaining exposure

It is critical to acquire accurate exposure data on cases and controls. If information collected from cases and controls is not of comparable quality, we are in for trouble. Since exposure data are assembled *after* outcomes are known, it is not difficult to imagine that such knowledge might influence the gathering of information. Both subjects and investigators may fall prey to bias that occurs when one looks backward.

Subject bias Many case-control studies rely on information supplied by the subjects themselves. But case and comparison subjects are apt to have considered the past rather differently. People who have unpleasant diseases are likely to have scrutinized past events with much greater vigor than nondiseased individuals. It is human nature to seek explanations for tragedies. So it should not surprise us that people who are beleaguered by illness or unpleasant outcomes have contemplated deeply what caused their problem and may have an overly detailed, even distorted picture of the past. This phenomenon is known as *selective recall*, or *recall bias*. An anecdote that illustrates the point occurred in the armed forces during World War II. Some savants hypothesized that aviators who had crashed their airplanes might have been accident-prone as youngsters. If this were true, it would certainly be important to know, so that these dangerous men might be identified and kept out of the cockpit. A case-control type of study was performed comparing flyers who had crashed their planes with a group of wreck-less pilots. Both groups were asked to report any accidents that occurred to them as children. Lo and behold, the flyers with the bad safety records emerged as several times more accident-prone than their colleagues. Hypothesis proven! Fortunately, wiser heads realized that the trauma of crashing an airplane might lead to self-indicting ruminations about the past. The experiment was repeated; this time the questions about accidents were asked of flyers as they came into the service, before any crashes had occurred. Freed of the problem of biased recall, investigators found that self-reported accident-proneness was not useful for predicting pilots who would have future accidents.

In an attempt to unravel the troubling mystery of sudden infant death syndrome (SIDS), British investigators created a case-control study to test the hypothesis that an infant's sleeping position is a risk factor.[13] For each case of SIDS identified, county health visitors were asked to select two infants from among their client load who lived in their neighborhood and were close to the same age as the case subjects. Parents of both groups were questioned about a host of social and medical factors, including the infant's habitual sleeping position and the position in which the child was sleeping at the time of the SIDS episode. It was found that 93 percent of SIDS cases compared to only 57 percent of controls slept in the prone position (i.e., on their stomachs). This difference translated to a strong association between sleeping habits and sudden death.

Critics countered that distraught parents of SIDS cases might have exhibited recall bias in reporting their infant's sleeping position.[14,15] The "inevitable guilt that follows a sudden infant death and the parents' consequent need to seem to have done everything possible to care for their baby"[14] means that parents might have overreported prone-position sleeping, which is considered by authorities, including child-care books, to be "safer" for babies.

Assessing subject bias Any evidence that researchers have checked on the memory of subjects should be welcome and is notice to the reader that authors are on their toes. Concerned about the possibilities of recall bias that had been suggested by others, investigators from Australia compared available data on infant sleeping positions that had been obtained both prospectively, as part of a large follow-up study, and after the fact using a case-control design.[16] The estimated increased risk of the prone sleeping position was similar for both studies, suggesting that the higher rate of prone-position sleeping reported by parents of SIDS victims was not simply a manifestation of recall bias.

In a case-control study evaluating estrogen therapy given to women to relieve menopausal symptoms and the subsequent risk of developing breast cancer,[17] the authors were aware that the history of drug use given by women who had breast cancer might be biased toward the recall of use of estrogens. This was especially likely in view of the substantial controversy the topic has generated in the lay press. The investigators took the additional trouble to review subjects' medical records to document estrogen use as well as to check records from major pharmacies in the community. Thus, three estimates of estrogen use were obtained. The researchers were able to show that recall bias did not seem to be playing a role. Estimates of the increased likelihood of breast cancer in high-dosage estrogen users were similar for the three data sources.

Alternate sources of data are not always available. Another way of assessing the possible role of recall bias is to note how cases respond to questions that are not related to the outcome. Some investigators will even include dummy items—questions they feel are unrelated to urinary tract infections, cancer, or angina—and see if there is a differential response rate between cases and controls. Case subjects who are exhibiting selective recall should overrespond and identify a large number of items as potentially related to the outcome. So a useful tip for the clinical reader is to take note of how specific the list of associated factors is. If cancer victims recall heavy utilization of five or six different medications, watch out! If only one of a large list of drugs or behaviors has a higher frequency in cases than controls, selective recall is probably less likely.

Although not all case-control studies are able to provide evidence that selective recall is not a problem, savvy investigators will at least be cognizant of the importance of this potential bias in their work and report any measures they took to try to master it. The intriguing topic of subject bias has been discussed in several thought-provoking reviews.[18,19]

Researcher bias   When investigators know the identity of case and comparison subjects and which exposures are risks they are seeking, objectivity is put to a strenuous test. It is difficult not to search medical records more thoroughly or question more diligently about exposure to asbestos in cases of fibrotic lung disease or about the consumption of artificial sweeteners among bladder cancer patients. And while such exuberance can be appreciated as an understandable human foible, readers need some assurance that researchers have attempted to guard against such potential bias.

In a classic case-control study of smoking and lung cancer published in 1950,[20] the study directors were concerned that interviewers' awareness of which patients had lung cancer might lead them to obtain unequal smoking histories. To test for possible bias, they conducted a substudy in which 100 patients with lung cancer and 186 patients with other chest diseases were interviewed by two nonmedical investigators who were unaware of the patients' diagnosis. When distributions of smoking histories for cases and controls in the main study and the substudy were compared, exposure rates were strikingly similar (see Fig. 3-1). It appeared, therefore, that interviewer bias was not a problem.

In a study that sought predictive factors in the social environment of patients who had Hodgkin's disease,[21] authors went to elegant lengths to demonstrate that information obtained from controls without cancer was similar to that provided by case patients with Hodgkin's. Interviewers were asked not only to rate the reliability of interviewees but also to record the amount of time spent talking with each subject. The research team was able to report that *information biases* did not appear to be responsible for differences found, since subject reliability rated as similar for both cases and controls and time spent in the interviews was almost identical, averaging 28.1 and 26.7 minutes for the two groups, respectively.

Nested case-control studies Sometimes fortune blesses investigators with a large cohort study that provides valid data from the past and a common population source for cases and controls. The result is a *nested case-control study*, or case control within a cohort. Two groups of researchers, both exploring the possible relationship between *Helicobacter pylori* infection and gastric carcinoma, have employed this design with good effect. In both instances, large cohorts had been assembled some 20 years earlier. Blood samples were taken and stored. The first cohort consisted of more than 7000 Japanese-American men who enrolled in the Honolulu Heart Study,[22] the second group was a

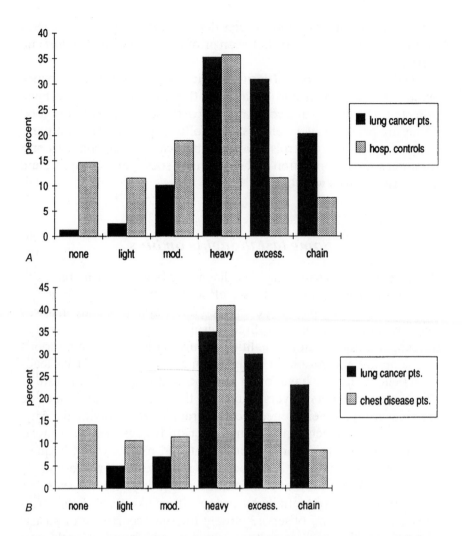

FIGURE 3-1 *A.* **Amount of smoking among 605 male patients with lung cancer and 780 general hospital control patients.** *B.* **Amount of smoking among 100 male patients with lung cancer and 186 male chest disease patients. (Adapted from Wynder and Graham.[20] Copyright 1950, American Medical Association. Reprinted by permission.)**

part of a Kaiser Permanente multiphasic health program.[23] By 1989, over 100 men from the Honolulu study and 200 from the Kaiser program had been diagnosed with gastric carcinoma. Age-matched controls were selected for each case and antibody titers to *H. pylori* were determined for each pair from the previously collected blood samples.

Patients with cancer in both studies demonstrated higher titers, indicating a positive association between prior infection with *H. pylori* and gastric cancer.

The nested case-control design is efficient in time and money, since outcomes are known and data from the past have already been collected. The quality and comparability of these data are usually good if they are products of a well-designed follow-up study. The comparability of cases and controls is also high because they come from a common source population and share many social, demographic, and health-risk factors with one another.

Some last thoughts on bias

We have discussed sampling bias, diagnostic bias, reporting bias, and recall bias. Other potential biases afflict the methodology. Bias can occur any time groups being compared differ systematically in a way that is related to the outcome. Study results may be upset when we fail to recognize important inequalities of information gathering, reporting, sampling, utilization, or observation between groups. Bias leads us to believe that we have found an important increase in the rate of childhood accidents in flyers who crash their planes when in fact we are measuring the heightened recall of traumatized individuals. Anytime a reader suspects that a group under study goes to doctors more, has more complete records kept, is watched more closely, is questioned more thoroughly, is subjected to more tests, or represents an unusual sub-group of a population, the possibility of bias exists. Patients who are on potentially hazardous drugs like steroids or estrogens are likely to be observed closely for the occurrence of gastric ulcers or uterine cancer, so these diseases are found at early presymptomatic stages that might go undetected in patients not on red-flag medication. Similarly, patients with diseases that have known risk factors or causes, such as emphysema or bladder cancer, may be questioned in greater detail about use of tobacco or artificial sweeteners than control subjects. A voluntary response bias can arise when case subjects who think they have been exposed to a potential carcinogen like arsenic or asbestos return mailed questionnaires at a higher rate than controls. Sackett has listed 35 variations on the bias theme.[24] The names and nuances are of less importance to clinicians than an understanding of the basic concept.

While readers should be vigilant for the multiple possible sources of bias, it is also well to retain a modicum of perspective. It is not reasonable to dismiss a study as unworthy simply because the possibility for bias exists. Often, when verification of bias (or non-bias) is sought, the information supplied by subjects or data collectors proves quite adequate to the task. Study results may quaver with the threat of biases, but often there is little damage done.

One must also remember that the problems that we have identified may operate in differing directions. Bias may create or accentuate an apparent difference between cases and controls, or it may hide one. A study that finds a strong relationship between coronary artery disease and smoking may include as cases subjects who are unlikely to have heart disease. But this dilution of cases with non-cases will *reduce* rather than *inflate* differences between groups. Results would be even more dramatic if our criterion of strict adherence to case definitions were followed. As critical readers, we must assess not only the potential for bias but also the likelihood of its occurrence and actual effect. Often the consequences are minimal if they exist at all.

SUMMARY

Once a study has been identified as a case-control design, ask the following:

1. What kind of population do the cases represent? Are they a valid representation of the disease or outcome in question or a subset of that population for whom responses are not typical? Have cases been carefully defined to represent a single disease entity or outcome, or are they a mixture of potentially unrelated conditions?

2. How like the case subjects are the controls? Are they drawn from a similar population, differing only in the absence of disease, or are there differences that might bear a relationship to the outcome of the study? If hospital controls are selected,

do their diseases bear a relationship to the exposure under study? Are controls likely to over- or underrepresent the exposure status of a general population? If community controls are used, have they been sampled so as to reflect the entire makeup of the community? Have investigators used techniques such as multiple control groups or matching in an effort to improve estimates of exposure among the non-diseased and make controls and cases as comparable as possible?

3. Have data on the exposure in question been accurately obtained from both cases and controls? Are subject or investigator biases creating or masking differences? Do researchers attempt to verify data using multiple sources?

4. Are other biases evident? Do we know more about cases because they have been under closer surveillance, have volunteered more information, or have been subjected to more extensive testing that control subjects?

Passing this critical barrage is a difficult task for a case-control study, but the methods used to conduct studies of this sort are continually improving. A critical look at studies for these common limitations of design may lead to the disquieting conclusion that a number of efforts are not credible. On the other hand, we should feel some joy that investigators are becoming increasingly facile with this challenging methodology and often succeed in providing useful information with maximum efficiency.

REFERENCES

1. Cole P: The evolving case-control study. *J Chron Dis* 32:15, 1979.
2. Hymes KB, Greene JB, Marcus A et al: Kaposi's sarcoma in homosexual men—A report of eight cases. *Lancet* 2:598, 1981.
3. Illegal fishing, editorial. *Lancet* 2:1268, 1981.
4. Hayden GF, Kramer MS, Horwitz RI: The case-control study: A practical review for the clinician. *JAMA* 247:326, 1982.
5. Cassano PA, Koepsell TD, Farwell JR: Risk of febrile seizures in childhood in relation to prenatal maternal cigarette smoking and alcohol intake. *Am J Epidemiol* 132:462, 1990.
6. Klebanoff MA: Invited commentary: The epidemiology of febrile sei-

zures, or the epidemiology of study participation. *Am J Epidemiol* 132:474, 1990.

7. Schlech WF III, Shands KN, Reingold AL et al: Risk factors for development of toxic shock syndrome: Association with a tampon brand. *JAMA* 248:835, 1982.

8. Harvey M, Horwitz RI, Feinstein AR: Toxic shock and tampons: Evaluation of the epidemiologic evidence. *JAMA* 248:840, 1982.

9. Hurwitz ES, Barrett MJ, Bregman D et al: Public Health Service study of Reye's syndrome and medications: Report of the main study. *JAMA* 257:1905, 1987.

10. MacMahon B, Yen S, Trichopoulos D et al: Coffee and cancer of the pancreas. *N Engl J Med* 304:630, 1981.

11. Silverman DT, Hoover RN, Swanson M, Hartge P: The prevalence of coffee drinking among hospitalized and population-based control groups. *JAMA* 249:1877, 1983.

12. Oleinick MS, Bahn AK, Eisenberg L, Lilienfeld AM: Early socialization experiences and intrafamilial environment: A study of psychiatric outpatient and control group children. *Arch Gen Psychiatry* 15:344, 1966.

13. Fleming PJ, Gilbert R, Azaz Y et al: Interaction between bedding and sleeping position in the sudden infant death syndrome: A population based case-control study. *Br Med J* 301:85, 1990.

14. Southall D, Stebbens V, Samuel M: Bedding and sleep position in the sudden infant death syndrome. *Br Med J* 301:492, 1990.

15. Wailoo MP, Peterson SA: Bedding and sleep position in the sudden infant death syndrome. *Br Med J* 301:492, 1990.

16. Dwyer T, Ponsonby AB, Newman NM, Gibbons LE: Prospective cohort study of prone sleeping position and sudden infant death syndrome. *Lancet* 2:1244, 1991.

17. Ross RK, Paganini-Hill A, Gerkins VR et al: A case-control study of menopausal estrogen therapy and breast cancer. *JAMA* 243:1635, 1980.

18. Coughlin SS: Recall bias in epidemiologic studies. *J Clin Epidemiol* 43:87, 1990.

19. Neugebauer R, Ng S: Differential recall as a source of bias in epidemiologic research. *J Clin Epidemiol* 43:1337, 1990.

20. Wynder EL, Graham EA: Tobacco smoking as a possible etiologic factor in bronchiogenic carcinoma: A study of six hundred and eighty-four proved cases. *JAMA* 143:329, 1950.

21. Gutensohn N, Cole P: Childhood social environment and Hodgkin's disease. *N Engl J Med* 304:135, 1981.

22. Nomura A, Stemmermann GN, Chyou PH et al: *Helicobacter pylori* and

gastric carcinoma among Japanese Americans in Hawaii. *N Engl J Med* 325:1132, 1991.

23. Parsonnet J, Friedman GD, Vandersteen DP et al: *Helicobacter pylori* infection and the risk of gastric carcinoma. *N Engl J Med* 325:1127, 1991.

24. Sackett DL: Bias in analytic research. *J Chronic Dis* 32:51, 1979.

CHAPTER FOUR

STUDY DESIGN: THE CROSS-SECTIONAL AND FOLLOW-UP APPROACHES

Had we but world enough and time,
This cohort study were no crime ....
But at my back I always hear
Time's winged chariot hurrying near;

—adapted from **ANDREW MARVELL**

$\mathcal{F}$rom studies that start with subjects who already have an outcome or disease, we will turn to evaluating designs that utilize the cross-sectional and follow-up approaches. As outlined in Chap. 2, these studies tackle the task of providing explanations by assembling groups of subjects that represent either a general, nondiseased population or people who share features we think might predispose them to a particular outcome. Subjects are classified by characteristics such as high cholesterol level, crowded living conditions, or occupational exposure to benzene. Then they are either simultaneously sorted by diseases they already have (for example, heart disease, mental illness, or leukemia) or followed for a period of time to see what develops.

In the cross-sectional, or prevalence, approach, it is all done at once, in a single slice of time. A population is chosen for study, a sample of the group is selected, and subjects are poked, probed, and pricked to find out how many have HIV antibody, what the adverse effects from hospital care may be, or how many physicians derive little satisfaction from their medical practices. At the same time, features or risk factors associated with these conditions are elicited. Often the purpose of the exercise is descriptive, to identify the magnitude and details of a health problem. Readers can alert themselves to the likelihood of encountering HIV-positive individuals among prenatal patients or meeting a disgruntled internist in Salt Lake City. On other occasions we are after explanations. Are symptoms of dizziness caused by hypoglycemia? What clinical features best identify patients with bacteremia, or which characteristics of hospitals are associated with poor medical care? Whether the goal is descriptive or explanatory, the same basic strategy applies. The design is schematized in Fig 4-1. Often subjects identified in these cross-sectional efforts go on to become the cohort or population of interest in a follow-up study. Pregnancies are

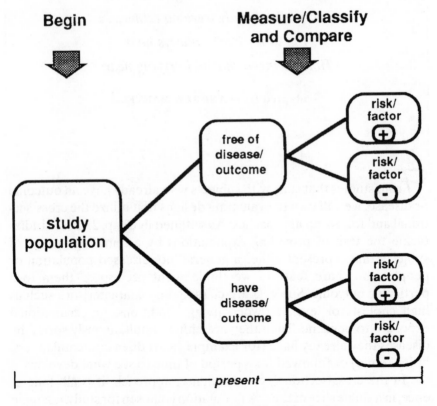

FIGURE 4-1 Cross-sectional study design.

monitored to find out how many infants become HIV infected, and internists are followed to see how many leave practice. Figure 4-2 recalls this approach. In this chapter, we will take a closer look at the contributions these study designs can make and learn some critical questions to ask each time one of the strategies is encountered.

CROSS-SECTIONAL DESIGNS

From the quick glance at cross-sectional designs offered in Chap. 2, one might infer that the approach is a country cousin to the more elegant follow-up design. It is true that prevalence studies are often conducted as screening and classification preambles to larger follow-up efforts. Before the incidence of heart disease in a community is studied, the population must be evaluated for current cardiac status and sorted by characteristics such as blood pressure, smoking, and cholesterol level. However, in a number of studies, the cross-sec-

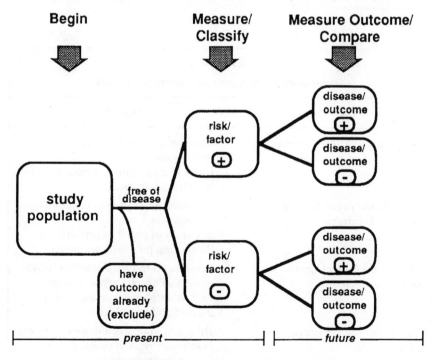

FIGURE 4-2 Follow-up study design.

tional design serves as the appetizer, main course, and dessert. In reviewing the designs utilized in articles from three of the most influential clinical journals, the Fletchers note that cross-sectional studies have become increasingly prevalent (pun intended).[1] In 1946, 24 percent of 151 journal articles surveyed were classified as cross-sectional in design, compared with 44 percent of articles published in 1976. This popularity indicates that the design has considerable flexibility and applicability beyond providing initial classification of patients for subsequent follow-up endeavors. Some of these applications are noted in Table 4-1.

The cross-sectional strategy shares some advantages of the case-control design. It is strong on efficiency. Conclusions are based on information collected at the same time, so investigators are not obliged to wait months or years in the anticipation of an outcome. Everything is done on the spot, often from information that is already at hand. Pharmacy records of antibiotics ordered in a community hospital are searched and usage is detailed according to medical specialty. Patients with juvenile rheumatoid arthritis are tested for histocompatibility antigens and compared by age and symptom patterns. Unfortunately,

---

• TABLE 4-1 •
Some uses of the cross-sectional approach

Use	Example
Evaluate a new test or the new application of an old one	Ultrasonography for deep venous thrombosis C-reactive protein to predict invasive streptococcal disease
Evaluate the predictive capability of clinical features	Relationship of physical examination to bacteremia Accuracy of rectal examination in diagnosing prostate carcinoma
Identify etiological agents or causative factors	*Salmonella*-induced diarrhea subsequent to church barbecue supper Lactose intolerance as cause of recurrent abdominal pain
Determine the prevalence of a problem	Drug use among health professionals Disabilities related to age among hospitalized elderly

cross-sectional studies also share frailties with their case-control cousins. These include subject selection and response/participation bias.

Subject selection

Population selection   The kinds of subjects that find their way into cross-sectional studies can have a major influence on results. Earlier we discussed generalizability as an issue that must be addressed in reviewing studies. It is important to know if the acne patients described as responding favorably to topical treatment with clindamycin are enough like patients we see that comparable therapeutic results may be expected, or that our patients on birth control pills share features with patients that an article describes as being at increased risk for pulmonary embolism. Sometimes a study offers a view of health risks or outcomes that is accurate for a very special group of patients but that lacks relevance for the practice of the typical clinician. A mismatch is particularly likely when the study population is drawn from a tertiary hospital or referral center. These patients often pass through a complex filter before reaching the meccas. White et al. created a model depicting the selection process that takes place before patients arrive at tertiary medical centers.[2] As Fig. 4-3 suggests, only a fraction

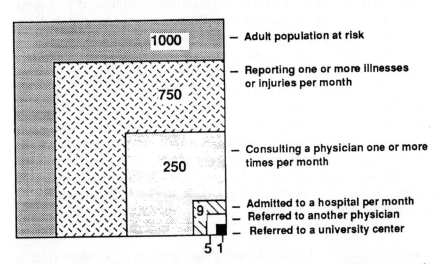

FIGURE 4-3   Monthly prevalence estimates of illness in the community and the roles of physicians, hospitals, and university medical centers in the provision of medical care (adults 16 years of age and over). (From White et al.[2] Reprinted by permission of the *New England Journal of Medicine*.)

of potential patients in a community become subjects for study in a referral center. Those who do are unlikely to be representative of the 999 folks back home. Information gathered on such highly selected patients can be misleading.

An example of population selection at work may be seen from comparing two studies on the etiology of low back pain. One of these reports comes from the Mayo Clinic,[3] a very special referral center, the other from a family-practice setting.[4] Investigators from each of these sites reviewed the cases of low back pain they had seen over a period of time and described the frequency with which herniated intervertebral disc disease was diagnosed. According to the Mayo Clinic, ruptured discs were responsible for 22 percent of cases of low back pain; in family practice, only 4.4 percent of low back pain sufferers were suspected of having disc problems, with only 2 of 140 cases reviewed (1.4 percent) actually confirmed by myelogram and surgically treated. The most likely factor contributing to the varying results is the dissimilarity in the study populations. Most patients who go to Mayo have been to at least one other doctor. Many less important back problems never get referred, so by the time patients reach the clinic, a higher proportion of the pool has more severe disease, such as herniated discs. Physicians in general practice take on all comers and see a greater percentage of less complicated problems. Their experience more accurately reflects the frequency of disc disease in a general population than does the Mayo report.

Surveys designed to determine the prevalence of human immunodeficiency virus (HIV) infection offer another illustration of the importance of population selection. "How many people are infected with HIV?" Estimates vary considerably, depending upon the population one surveys.[5] If one samples clinics that treat sexually transmitted diseases, methadone treatment centers, or prisons, the estimate of infected individuals is very different from results obtained from military recruits, Red Cross blood donors, or applicants for marriage licenses. Table 4-2 gives some idea of the variety of estimates obtained from different populations.

Sample selection Once an author has chosen a population, it is important to find out who within the group becomes a study subject. There are a variety of ways authors can select samples. They may attempt to enroll every eligible subject in the study. That is fine for small populations, but with larger groups, it is not feasible. One

• TABLE 4-2 •
Seroprevalence of human immunodeficiency virus in different populations

Population	Positives/1000
Homosexual/bisexual men in San Francisco	490
Intravenous drug users in San Francisco	100
Nevada prison inmates	18
Massachusetts newborns	2.0
U.S. military recruits	1.5
Red Cross blood donors	0.2

SOURCE: Centers for Disease Control.[5]

approach to dealing with bigger populations is systematic sampling, which involves selecting every second or third patient who is available or picking only patients with even numbers as the last digits of their medical records. Another technique is random sampling, in which a portion of available patients is chosen by selection of random numbers or drawing from a hat. This assures each member of the population an equal chance of being included in the study. The question that readers must ask is whether the sampling technique employed has guarded against the selection of a biased or unrepresentative sample. Authors may report that patients were selected at random when, in fact, strict randomizing techniques, such as using a random-numbers table or other unbiased procedure, were not used. Used colloquially, the term *random selection* means unplanned or haphazard sampling. It suggests that the authors had no sampling plan in mind but simply took a convenience sample of subjects to enroll in the study. This is not good enough. Very unrepresentative samples of subjects can be obtained when laissez-faire sampling techniques are used.

Let us look at an early study on outpatient blood cultures as an aid to diagnosing the cause of fever in children.[6] This is a good example of a cross-sectional design that seeks evidence for the utility of the application of a test (blood cultures) to clarify a clinical problem (fever of unknown origin). All febrile children attending a walk-in clinic during a 3-month period were eligible for study. Blood cultures were obtained from these children to ascertain the prevalence of bacteremia, and subjects were simultaneously cross-classified by characteristics such as degree of fever, age, and white blood cell count to augment the clinician's predictive power (see Table 4-3).

The authors do well in clearly defining fever as a "rectal temperature of 38.3°C or higher or an oral temperature of 37.8°C or higher," but they report as their sampling technique only that "physicians of the pediatric service were requested to obtain a blood culture from febrile patients." It turns out that during the 3-month study period, 2059 children who met the fever criteria visited the clinic. Of these, only 415, or 20 percent, actually had blood cultures obtained. In other words, only one-fifth of eligible patients were included. With no more information than we have at hand regarding the sampling procedure, can we assume that the children included represent the entire population in an unbiased fashion? Probably not. Children on whom blood cultures were done are likely to have been kids who worried physicians because they appeared to have a toxic condition; that is, they were suspected of having a bacterial infection such as pneumonia or meningitis. Youngsters who appeared to have benign febrile illnesses, such as roseola or viral gastroenteritis, would be less promising candidates

---

· **TABLE 4-3** ·

Factors associated with bacteremia in febrile children

Factor	Percent of patients with positive blood cultures
Fever	
Less than 38.9°C	0.9
38.9 to 39.9°C	6.6
40.0°C or greater	8.0
Age	
Less than 12 months	6.7
13 to 24 months	4.6
25 months or greater	2.7
White blood cell count	
Less than 10,000/mm^3	1.1
10,000 to 19,900/mm^3	6.1
At or above 20,000/mm^3	11.6

SOURCE: Modified from McGowan et al.[6]

for culture. Any estimate of the frequency of bacteremia in this selected sample is probably an overestimate of the likelihood of positive blood cultures among the general population of febrile children. The results may give us an idea of how often bacteria can be isolated from the blood of very sick youngsters, but without a clear description of the selection that went on, we have no way of generalizing the data. Had the authors provided us with comparative information about the clinical condition of the patients sampled and those excluded, the data they provide might be more useful.

The question of HIV prevalence provides another example of sampling problems. To estimate the occurrence of HIV infection among university students in the United States, blood samples from 19 universities across the country were collected and tested for antibodies to HIV.[7] Of almost 17,000 specimens collected, 30, or 0.2 percent, had detectable HIV antibodies. This rate of 1 positive for 500 students tested was acknowledged to be lower than rates found among high-risk groups, but it was greater than the prevalence of 0.15 percent found in civilian applicants for military service.[5] The popular press reported on the study findings and extrapolated results to estimate that 25,000 college students across the nation may be infected with HIV.

But, the sampling techniques used in this project raise serious questions about the validity of such claims. In an attempt to maintain confidentiality, the serosurvey was conducted not on a random sample of students at the 19 universities but on a *convenience sample* of blood specimens that were collected at university health centers in the course of clinical care. While such a procedure may be desirable from the privacy perspective, it creates an unsatisfactory sample. We know nothing about the study participants except that they visited the health services and had conditions that clinicians felt required a blood test. It is likely that some made clinic visits related to sexually transmitted diseases, and some may have been concerned that they had been exposed to HIV. Students who visit health centers and have blood taken are not representative of the general student body.

Response/participation bias

Even when a population is carefully chosen and samples are selected to provide accurate estimates of that population, studies can suffer if subjects do not cooperate. Lack of participation may occur for a host of reasons. Subjects may have moved or cannot be contacted, they may be too ill to participate or even have died, or they may decline for a variety of personal reasons. The chief concern is, of course, that people who agree to answer questions and submit to blood tests differ from those who do not. If systematic dissimilarities between participants and nonparticipants are related to the outcomes we are attempting to measure, results may be distorted.

An example borrowed from the social science literature offers a dramatic illustration. A survey of U.S. women that found wide coverage in the popular literature proclaimed that a large proportion of women were deeply dissatisfied with their relationships with men.[8] The report was based on results of 100,000 questionnaires that were distributed to a variety of groups across the country, including women's organizations, church groups, and counseling and walk-in centers for women and families. While the magnitude of the survey is impressive, the issue is not the number of questionnaires distributed but the proportion of those returned. In this case, only 4500 responses, or 4.5 percent of those distributed, were returned. This is a very low rate and, as critics pointed out, is unlikely to give an accurate representation of the 100,000 women queried.[9] "Responses usually come disproportionately from those who are agitated by, or concerned about an issue. It is thus likely that the small minority of women who responded would be heavily drawn from those who were dissatisfied with their personal relationships with men."[9]

At the start of a follow-up study of coronary heart disease and stroke among men of Japanese ancestry who were living in Honolulu, 73 percent of approximately 11,000 eligible men agreed to participate and submit to a baseline physical examination.[10] That left almost 3000 nonparticipants. Fortunately, investigators had also distributed a mailed questionnaire requesting information on certain biological and lifestyle characteristics. Because this had been returned by 60 percent of men who subsequently declined participation in the larger study, certain features of participants and nonparticipants could be compared. It was discovered that the two groups differed significantly in several important respects. Participants were more likely to be married, to have a high school education, to have been previously hospitalized, and to be nonsmokers. When mortality figures for the two groups were assessed 14 years later, participants, with their lower risk profiles, had significantly lower mortality than nonparticipants.

Unfortunately, because they are nonresponders, we often lack information on nonparticipants that can be used to assess such bias.

Investigators should share what information they have on the comparability of respondents and nonrespondents. Supplying readers with the response or participation rate is a minimum requirement. How high the rate should be to be considered acceptable is a matter of debate. Rates in excess of 80 percent are considered very good by most, and those below 40 percent as quite suspicious. Obviously, even relatively small groups of nonresponders may differ in important ways from their parent populations, as the Honolulu Heart Study example illustrates. Any sort of demographic or risk-factor information that authors can supply to clarify the situation is helpful. Details as to why folks declined participation can also be of use.

Time-order relationships

Cross-sectional studies fall prey to a chicken-and-egg dilemma. Since information related to a subject's outcome is collected at the same time as data on the possible causative or predictive factor, it is not always clear which comes first. Does the attribute or characteristic really lead to the effect or disease, or does the outcome in some way predispose people to acquire factors or characteristics that appear to be predictive?

Cross-sectional studies that explore childhood obesity offer an example. A common finding has been that children who are overweight are less active than their normal-weight contemporaries. The conclusion drawn from these reports is that children who have low levels of activity are more likely to become obese. But again, antecedent-consequent relationships are muddied when data on causes and effects are collected at the same time. It is also plausible that children with weight problems have difficulty getting around and are inactive because of their obesity rather than that they are fat because they are inactive.

The time-order problem is a frailty which cross-sectional design shares with case-control efforts. An example comes from the literature on childhood lead poisoning. While severe lead intoxication is known to cause seizures and encephalopathy, the effect of lower levels of chronic lead exposure on neurologic development has been an important research question. Investigators from New York hypothesized that lead intoxication might be an important cause of hyperactivity among children.[11] To test their idea, they assembled several samples of children from a pediatric outpatient clinic. Some of these children carried the diagnosis of hyperactivity, some had been diagnosed and treated as having lead poisoning, and some were nonhyperactive comparisons. The strategy was simply to measure blood and urine lead levels among these children to see if differences could be found among the groups. The investigators found that for children identified as being hyperactive "without a presumed cause," lead levels were substantially higher than for the nonhyperactive controls. They conclude that these increased lead levels make it "conceivable that one consequence of this constant minimal poisonous assault is hyperactivity." However, there is an important reservation one must raise about this interpretation. As the authors themselves query, "might the lead levels recorded be a consequence of the child's hyperactivity rather than a hyperactivity cause?" It is a good question. Lead poisoning may indeed cause hyperactive behavior. However, it is also known that hyperactive children tend to have high rates of other untoward behaviors, such as pica, the ingestion of nonfood substances. Children who are hyperactive may eat more lead paint than the comparison group, so the evidence of lead accumulation in the body becomes a reflection of the hyperactive behavior rather than a cause of it.

Sequential cross-sectional studies

Cross-sectional studies are frequently repeated at various time intervals, then combined to depict trends that alert us to the progress we are making on solving health problems or the need to increase our efforts. Large sequential cross-sectional surveys show us that rates of smoking are declining in the population, seat-belt use is reluctantly increasing, and measles immunization rates have fallen to embarrassing levels. This is useful information. And for large, well-constructed surveys like many conducted by the National Center for Health Statistics, the information is quite dependable. But trends are built upon repeated cross-sectional studies which assume that representative sampling of the same parent population takes place. If the composition of the reference population changes over time, if sampling is altered, or if patterns of response change, apparent trends in seat-belt use may be due to quirks of method rather than health behavior. The AIDS literature again provides instruction.

Investigators from the New York State Department of Health provided seropositivity information for a number of New York State HIV testing sites over a period of several years.[12] Data on the numbers of individuals tested and the percentage with positive tests over four sequential time periods are shown in Table 4-4.

If one were presented with only the data from the top rows of the table, the trend would appear to be encouraging. The data show that the number of individuals tested grew substantially, while the percent with positive results fell. One might conclude that infection with HIV is on the wane and the epidemic in decline. However, the authors provide additional information that dampens any such optimism. When questionnaire data obtained from those tested are added to the table, substantial changes in the composition of the groups studied in the sequential periods are evident. The proportion of individuals with high-risk behaviors for HIV infection or who were experiencing symptoms fell over time. Greater numbers of lower-risk individuals sought testing. The fall in HIV seroprevalence cannot be attributed to declining rates of infection without accounting for the dramatic changes in the population undergoing testing.

FOLLOW-UP STUDIES

The follow-up, or cohort, design is generally considered to be the crème de la crème of observational methodologies. It is unencumbered by many of the problems that beset the case-control and cross-sectional approaches. Since data are gathered prospectively rather than from rooting through records of the past, they may be collected

· Table 4-4 ·			
Serologic testing for human immunodeficiency virus over four periods of time			
	1/86–6/86	7/86–12/86	1/87–6/87	7/87–12/87
Number tested	2127	2374	4989	7602
Percent positive	14.5	13.6	5.7	4.2
%male	72.5	66.4	57.8	56.3
%symptomatic	17.7	16.4	8.0	8.0
%IV drug user	5.0	14.9	10.9	10.8
%homo/bisexual	42.9	39.7	26.1	24.6

SOURCE: Modified from Grabau and Morse.[12]

in a comprehensive and uniform fashion. No need to worry whether height and weight were recorded in the chart or whether blood pressure was accurately measured. Investigators can set up the rules before they begin. Nor is recall bias a problem, since patients are not being asked to recall events of the past but will be followed into the future to see which outcomes develop. Time-order relationships are also made clear, as patients are classified by characteristics before the disease or outcome becomes manifest. Activity levels of children of normal weight can be documented before they are followed to see who develops obesity. It is all much tidier, there is much more control over the quality of the data, and there is greater clarity in the sequence of events. Had we, as Andrew Marvell suggests, no constraints of resources and unlimited time, it would be the ideal strategy. Unfortunately, substantial costs are likely to be incurred in following large populations, and "time's winged chariot" does, in fact, press us.

Follow-up studies are also not without their methodological weak points. In addition to that persistent plague, population selection, there are three other afflictions that we have not examined thus far: loss to follow-up, changes in subject characteristics, and surveillance bias.

Selection

Follow-up designs are susceptible to selection problems. An elegant illustration comes from the literature on febrile convulsions in children. In a typical case, a toddler 1 to 2 years of age will be bundled to the emergency room by frantic parents. The child seemed fine, they report, until he suddenly fell to the floor, eyes rolled back, in a generalized tonic-clonic convulsion. The seizure lasted for only a few minutes, and not until the aftermath did the parents realize the child was febrile to 104°F. This is a horrifying experience for parents. When the initial anxiety abates, their most immediate concerns are, "Will it happen again?" and "Does this mean my child has epilepsy?" Good questions! Just the kind requiring a good natural history or follow-up study to answer. The answer, however, is very much dependent on the kind of population whose natural history is assessed. A study from Edinburgh, for example, followed 200 children admitted to a teaching hospital with the diagnosis of febrile convulsion.[13] The researchers found that almost 17 percent of these children had subsequent nonfebrile recurrences, which is quite a large number. However, if the response to parents about epilepsy is based on a Greek study,[14] febrile seizure patients will have a 65 percent chance of having later nonfebrile seizures. For those who find this prospect much too distressing, Nelson and Ellenberg give an overall risk of nonfebrile recurrences of only 3 percent.[15] That's certainly more encouraging! With such a wide variety of results, all coming from reputable journals, how do we know whom to believe?

In fact, all these studies may be right. They may all accurately portray the risk of recurrent seizures for the particular population they are observing. Readers must decide how the groups of patients reported compare with those they will be seeing. In this particular situation, the Scottish study reports on children who were hospitalized at a large medical center, the Greek study describes patients referred to a special developmental evaluation center, and Nelson's patients come from a cohort of 54,000 newborn infants from 11 U.S. cities who were followed for some years to detect neurological abnormalities. Ethnic differences notwithstanding, the broad population sample best reflects the kind of patients most doctors encounter and suggests that for most children who experience febrile convulsions, the risk of subsequent, nonfebrile attacks is small.

To confirm their impression that sample selection plays an important role in the results one finds, Ellenberg and Nelson made some further comparisons.[16] They reviewed 26 published articles that estimated the likelihood of nonfebrile seizures for children with febrile fits and classified findings by two categories of study populations. One group was composed of clinic-based studies—those that followed patients who came from hospital clinics or specialty referral units. The other group contained population-based studies—where a clearly defined general population was used. The comparative rates of recurrence are depicted in Fig. 4-4. Estimates for clinic-based studies are highly variable, ranging up to 75 percent; figures derived from population-based studies are much lower and remarkably consistent at about 3 percent.

Every study will have its own population of subjects, and each will have limits of generalizability. Readers must decide how closely subjects described in the study mirror patients they will be treating. Good authors will help in this task. Readers have a right to expect a reasonable amount of information about patients described in any study. What are their demographic characteristics? Where do they come from? Have they been referred from other medical-care facilities or have they come on their own? What is the reputation of the facility where the patients were gathered? Is it known to attract certain kinds

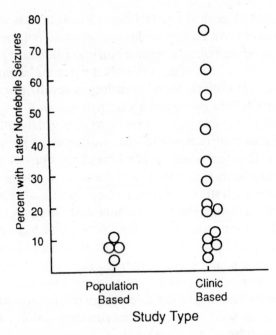

FIGURE 4-4 Percentage of children who experienced nonfebrile seizures after one or more febrile seizures, in population-based (left) and clinic-based (right) studies. (From Ellenberg and Nelson.[16] Copyright 1980, American Medical Association. Reprinted by permission.)

of patients with certain kinds of illnesses? Is it a specialty clinic? Only armed with this information can the reader address the problem of external validity or generalizability. If our patients are very unlike those being described in the study, we may be justified in feeling some reluctance to embrace the author's conclusions.

Loss to Follow-up

No matter how carefully one's sample is chosen, no matter how elegantly representative of the population, if subjects are lost to follow-up, we are in trouble. The biggest single problem of follow-up-design investigations is the loss of valuable information through attrition. Subjects change addresses, fail to respond to questionnaires, decide they no longer wish to participate, or just plain cannot be located. Dropouts are unfortunate, not simply because they reduce the numbers of subjects observed but also because the reasons they become lost to follow-up may be related to the outcomes under study. That adds another source of bias.

An illustration comes from the report of a study on the likelihood that women who lose babies will become depressed during the 6-month postpartum period.[17] Study subjects included women who had had a stillborn infant or whose baby died in the first 7 days of life. A complete sample of mothers who lost babies was taken for a year in an entire English county. For each of these, a comparison subject was chosen from all the mothers residing in the same locale who had had live births in that year. The authors matched the cases and controls by place and time of delivery. It is worth recalling here that while the authors speak of these comparison mothers as controls and refer to perinatal death subjects as cases, they are not utilizing a case-control design. The action of the study is forward and perinatal death is not the outcome but a potential risk factor for postpartum depression. The authors are forced to sample from the total pool of comparison patients, since to have included all live births would have created an extremely large cohort.

Questionnaires were given out at 2 days, 6 days, 6 weeks, and 6 months postpartum, asking women to report on symptoms related to depression. When returned questionnaires were tallied and evaluated for the presence of depressive symptomatology, a rather surprising finding emerged. "At 6 months, postpartum depression was just as common in women aged under 24 whose babies had survived as in women of the same age whose babies had died." This revelation is certainly contrary to what one would expect. Unfortunately, diligent as the authors were in their attempts to keep track of the women they enrolled in the study, not everyone responded to the questionnaire. And there is reason to believe that this loss to follow-up was biased. The authors note that "compared with the control group, fewer of the women whose babies had died responded to the six-month questionnaire." It also happens that in both groups the nonresponse rate was "more than twice as high" for women whose day-2 depression scores were high than for those whose rating indicated no depression. This information has some sticky implications. If women failed to respond to questionnaires because they were depressed, the unexpectedly low rate of postpartum depression among women who lost babies is an artifact of biased follow-up. These women are depressed—so depressed they are not up to completing and returning a depression inventory.

Subject loss is the bane of the follow-up study. A questionnaire is sent to patients asking them to report their satisfaction with a recent visit to the clinic. Only 50 percent respond. Are those who do not respond failing to do so because they are angry and dissatisfied or because they are pleased with the service and have no complaints? A study is designed to follow respiratory function of workers who have occupational exposure to cotton dust. A substantial number of workers cannot be located 10 years later, when it is time to evaluate their pulmonary status. Is there anything special about the group that cannot be found? Have they all changed jobs because of respiratory incapacity? Have they moved to Arizona so they can breathe? The possibility that attrition in studies is due to the factors being explored is substantial.

There are several ways that investigators can deal with the follow-up problem. Canny readers should check behind the author to see if this homework has been performed.

1. Has the investigator made every effort to track down lost subjects? Repeat mailings, telephone contacts, or home visits give evidence that investigators have been diligent in their efforts to locate wayward subjects and suggest concern about attrition. The authors of the report on perinatal death and depression get positive marks for their effort.[18] Second mailings were sent to all nonresponders to the first letter, and health visitors were sent to homes of those who failed to respond to the second mailing. Losses still occurred.

2. Do authors report the rate of follow-up loss and explore the possibility of biased attrition? Recognizing that some loss is inevitable, authors should detail the extent of the problem and offer information on characteristics of the nonrespondents. Authors should be able to provide demographic features, such as age, sex, and some initial classifying information like responses to the first depression scale. The more information indicating that the lost sheep are similar to those in the fold, the more comfortable we may feel that an important attrition bias is not influencing results. Any follow-up study that fails to offer information on losses should be viewed with skepticism.

3. Another technique for characterizing nonrespondents or dropouts is to spend some additional effort to contact a representative sample of this total group. This may be a difficult task, since

initial efforts at contact have been unsuccessful; but the effort expended in attacking a small sample may reward the investigator with important information about the characteristics of these lost subjects.

Change in habits

Although the follow-up design appears to avoid the messy business of relying on the memories of subjects to catalog habits and exposures of the past, other snares await the best laid plans. Subjects can change their habits. Smokers quit smoking, the inactive take up jogging, and dieters stop using saccharine. When investigators rely on initial categorizations of smoking activity and use of artificial sweeteners, they may find themselves misclassifying subjects. People thought to be at high risk may alter their life-style or reduce their exposure to a drug or environmental contaminant. Those who are thought to be at low risk may begin snacking on potato chips or start work in an asbestos factory. If only small numbers of subjects change their roles in an unselected way, there is not much problem; if many people switch, it can be trouble. In the time it takes to follow the natural history of a group of people, many uncontrolled outside events can occur. A community health-education campaign may induce subjects to stop smoking or a national fad such as jogging may overtake even the most sedentary of the citizenry. Patients may read in the newspaper about the dangerous side effects of a drug they have been taking and decide to discontinue the medication. There is not a great deal investigators can do to control this phenomenon, but they can periodically reexamine subjects and update classifications. Readers should look for evidence that authors are alert to the issue and reexamine their cohort to see whether habits or exposures have changed.

Surveillance bias

Another bias in follow-up studies can occur if there is unequal surveillance of subjects being compared. This problem is shared by all the observational designs and occurs any time one group of subjects get scrutinized or examined more closely than others. A case in point is a follow-up study that describes antecedents of child abuse and neglect among premature infants.[18] Investigators collected extensive informa-

tion on 255 families who had infants admitted to the newborn inten-
sive-care unit of a university medical center. A "psychosocial risk
inventory" was created to help identify children who might be subsequent victims of child abuse. Included in the inventory was information such as adequacy of child spacing, social isolation, major life stress,
adequacy of child-care arrangements, and financial status. Each family
was scored and categorized as being at high or low psychosocial risk.
The authors found that after a follow-up period of 6 to 19 months, 10
of 41 infants (24 percent) assigned to the high-risk group were reported to be abused or neglected, compared with none of the infants
categorized as being at low psychosocial risk.

That is an impressive difference and suggests that the psychosocial
scoring system has great utility. Unfortunately a misstep in design
opens the way for significant surveillance bias. Infants who were
classified as high-risk on the basis of their inventory scores were
identified to social service agencies at the time of discharge from the
hospital. While this may have been desirable practice from the view-
point of supporting families in need of help, it seriously interferes with
the ability to give an unbiased assessment of the value of the scoring
system. Identifying the infants as at high risk for abuse also puts them
at high risk of close surveillance and at high risk for being reported for
abuse and neglect. It is like examining one group of histological
specimens under low-power scan and another group under oil immer-
sion. The closer you look, the more you find. Reading that evidence
of neglect included "leaving infants unattended at home, failing to
comply with routine immunizations, and failing to provide adequate
nutrition" suggests that differential surveillance is contributing to the
findings. Low-risk kids are probably also being left unattended—but
nobody is watching.

SUMMARY

Having come across a study design you identify as being a cross-sectional or follow-up approach, consider the following:

1. How is the study population selected? Do subjects come
   from a referral center, a general medical practice, or the

community at large? Are there special features or characteristics of patients that would select them for membership in
this particular population? Are they older, sicker, or richer,
or do they have more severe manifestations of a given disease?
Have they already come through selective filters in the medical
system? Do the authors provide sufficient information for
you to identify the population and judge its similarity to your
own?

2. Are procedures for sampling within this population clearly
    defined? Can you tell exactly how individual subjects were
    picked? Were they chosen in a manner that avoids selection
    bias? Do authors provide evidence that subjects who are
    eligible but not included in the study are similar to those that
    have been selected? Do authors acknowledge the potential
    for selection bias and give evidence of safeguards used to
    avoid it or demonstrate that the problem has not affected
    results?

3. Is participation or subject response bias occurring? Have au-
    thors included the participation or response rate in their re-
    sults? Has an attempt been made to characterize nonpartici-
    pants? Are they angrier, happier, or more health-conscious
    than those who agreed to the study? Are differences in these
    characteristics related to outcomes and likely to bias results?

4. When a cross-sectional approach is utilized, are time-order
    relationships clear? If subjects are simultaneously classified by
    behaviors or potentially causative characteristics and the ef-
    fects or outcomes, is cause and effect implied when the se-
    quence of events is not clear? Is it likely that the characteristic
    really leads to the outcome, or could people who have certain
    diseases secondarily acquire characteristics that appear caus-
    ative?

5. If a follow-up design is utilized, is there loss to follow-up? Are
    authors careful to detail the methods used to follow subjects
    and provide information about subjects who stay? Are these
    nonrespondents or dropouts likely to bias results? Are reasons
    for attrition likely to be related to outcomes under study? Did
    subjects fail to answer because they were depressed or had left
    town because they could not breathe?

6. Did subjects change habits or exposures during the course of study? Have those believed to be at high risk initially changed their status by altering lifestyle, occupation, or drug intake? Do authors periodically reexamine their cohorts to see if habits have changed?

7. Is surveillance bias occurring? Are the groups being compared being observed with equal intensity? Or is high-powered scrutiny being applied to certain subjects, which may bias results?

REFERENCES

1. Fletcher RH, Fletcher SW: Clinical research in general medical journals: A 30-year perspective. *N Engl J Med* 301:180, 1979.
2. White KL, Williams TF, Greenberg BG: The ecology of medical care. *N Engl J Med* 265:885, 1961.
3. Ghormley RK: An etiology study of backache and sciatic pain. *Proceedings of the Staff Meetings of the Mayo Clinic* 26:457, 1951.
4. Barton JE, Haight RO, Marsland DW, Temple TE Jr: Low back pain in the primary care setting. *J Fam Pract* 3:363, 1976.
5. Centers for Disease Control: Human immunodeficiency virus infection in the United States: A review of current knowledge. *MMWR* 36(suppl S6):22, 1987.
6. McGowan JE, Jr, Bratton L, Klein JO, Finland M: Bacteremia in febrile children seen in a "walk-in" pediatric clinic. *N Engl J Med* 288:1309, 1973.
7. Gayle HD, Keeling RP, Garcia-Tunon M, et al: Prevalence of the human immunodeficiency virus among university students. *N Engl J Med* 323:1538, 1990.
8. Wallis C, McDowell J: Back off, buddy. *Time* 68, 1987.
9. Smith TW: Sex counts: A methodological critique of Hite's *Women in Love*, in Turner CF, Miller HG, Moses LE (eds): *AIDS, Sexual Behavior, and Intravenous Drug Use*. Washington, D.C., National Academy Press, 1989.
10. Benfante R, Reed D, McLean C, Kagan A: Response bias in the Honolulu heart program. *Am J Epidemiol* 130:1088, 1989.
11. David O, Clark J, Voeller K: Lead and hyperactivity. *Lancet* 2:900, 1972.
12. Grabau JC, Morse DL: Seropositivity for HIV at alternate sites. *JAMA* 260:3128, 1988.
13. Wallace SJ: Spontaneous fits after convulsions with fever. *Arch Dis Child* 52:192, 1977.

14. Gregoriades AD: A medical and social survey of 231 children with seizures. *Epilepsia* 13:13, 1972.
15. Nelson KB, Ellenberg JH: Predictors of epilepsy in children who have experienced febrile seizures. *N Engl J Med* 295:1029, 1976.
16. Ellenberg JH, Nelson KB: Sample selection and the natural history of disease: Studies of febrile seizures. *JAMA* 243:1337, 1980.
17. Clarke M, Williams AJ: Depression in women after perinatal death. *Lancet* 1:916, 1979.
18. Hunter RS, Kilstrom N, Kraybill EN, Loda F: Antecedents of child abuse and neglect in premature infants: A prospective study in a newborn intensive care unit. *Pediatrics* 61:629, 1978.

CHAPTER FIVE

Study Design: The Experimental Approach

I took 12 patients in the scurvy ... two of these were ordered each a quart of cider ... Two others took 25 gutts of elixer vitriol ... two took two spoonfuls of vinegar ... two were put under a course of sea-water ... two others had each two oranges and one lemon ... two took the bigness of a nutmeg three-times-a-day ....

JAMES LIND, A Treatise of the Scurvy

$\mathcal{L}$et us now sing the praises of the controlled trial! Although its ancestry certainly dates back to the eighteenth century, when James Lind fed 12 British sailors everything from seawater and vinegar to oranges (not limes) in an attempt to treat scurvy, wide acceptance of the experimental strategy is a recent occurrence. The British trials on the chemotherapy of tuberculosis performed in the late 1940s by many accounts mark the birth of the modern fascination with the controlled trial. The controlled trial represents the only study design available for clinical researchers that approximates the laboratory experiment. Most noted as a recipe for comparing drug therapies, the technique has evolved into a tool for evaluating a wide variety of clinical problems. Examples include the use of the controlled trial to compare methods of childbirth, to study medical versus surgical treatment of coronary artery disease, and to assess relaxation and meditation as a means of reducing high blood pressure. The scope of the design has broadened to include what are, strictly speaking, nonclinical areas of concern, such as health services, education, and health administration. Trials have been created to evaluate the efficacy of nurse practitioners compared with physicians and to judge the effectiveness of campaigns promoting the use of seat belts. There are a growing number of aficionados who would subject every therapeutic maneuver to the scrutiny of the controlled trial before it was loosed on the public.

Certainly, after dealing with the frustrating biases of the round-about strategies of case-control and follow-up observational studies, the controlled trial presents a refreshing, direct approach. The many difficulties of studying populations in their free-living state appear to be obviated by the planned comparisons of drugs or surgical techniques, health-education programs, or administrative innovations that are possible with the controlled trial design. Life for researchers is much simpler when they have some control over interventions. Nevertheless, there are chinks in the armor of the controlled trial that medical readers must know about. We will look at four major areas of methodologic concern. The first of these has to do with entry criteria and how people get into the study. Next, we will scrutinize the intervention or treatment itself: whether it is reproducible, practical, and free of bias. The pitfalls of selecting a comparison population is a third area of concern, with some problems reminiscent of the case-control and follow-up designs. Finally, we will explore an area that is unique to the controlled trial, that of subject allocation, and see how bias can occur when subjects are placed into experimental groups. For those who become intrigued with the subject, excellent commentaries are available from Hill,[1] Sackett,[2] Louis and Shapiro,[3] and Chalmers et al.[4]

SUBJECTS: WHO GETS IN

The study population

As we have seen in discussing other study designs, the people an investigator chooses to study make a big difference. If relaxation therapy truly lowers blood pressure in a middle-class private practice, will it also work in an inner-city clinic? Will a new learning program developed for medical students at a large midwestern medical school be transferable to a small school on the east coast? Experimental studies are just as susceptible to population-selection problems as are observational designs.

An example comes from the literature evaluating the use of single doses of antibiotics for the treatment of urinary tract infections.[5] The goal of these experiments was to improve therapy for women with cystitis by demonstrating that a single 3-g dose of amoxicillin was as effective as the conventional therapy of 10 days of the same antibiotic. If single-dose therapy proved effective, thousands of practitioners and patients who were confronted with this common problem would benefit. The investigators went to some lengths to differentiate between women with cystitis or lower-tract infection and those who had pyelonephritis or more serious upper-tract disease. Patients were excluded if they had temperatures greater than 38°C, rigors, or flank pain, or if they appeared toxic, so—clinically—they all appeared to have cystitis. Further, a special fluorescent antibody-coated bacterial assay was performed on urine specimens obtained from each subject. The presence of antibody-coated bacteria suggests tissue invasion of the kidneys and was used as an indicator of upper-tract infection; non-antibody-coated bacteria were taken to indicate a superficial infection of the bladder.

As the authors suspected, the success of single-dose amoxicillin varied with the presence or absence of antibody coating (see Table 5-1). Investigators found that single-dose therapy was just as effective

• TABLE 5-1 •

Response of urinary tract infections, defined by the results of the antibody-coated bacteria assay, to single-dose and conventional therapy with amoxicillin

Assay result	Therapy[a]	No. of patients	No. of relapses[b]
Negative	Single-dose	22	0
Negative	Conventional	21	0
Positive	Conventional	18	9

[a]Single dose = 3 g; conventional = 250 mg q.i.d.
[b]One week after completion of therapy.

SOURCE: Modified from Fang et al.[5]

as the standard 10-day course for women who had lower-tract infections. All 22 patients who had non-antibody-coated bacteria and were given single-dose therapy showed symptomatic improvement within 2 days. Women who had lower-tract disease and were given conventional therapy had similar good results. However, for 18 patients whose infections were caused by antibody-coated bacteria, results were much less encouraging. Relapse rates were high even after conventional treatment. With almost a third of patients who appeared clinically to have uncomplicated cystitis turning out to be unsuitable candidates for single-dose treatment, the value of the new therapy for clinicians is questionable at best.

A subsequent paper by the same group of investigators supplied further insight into the problem.[6] The original study population had been selected from ambulatory patients of the Massachusetts General Hospital, a well-known big-city referral center. To add to the experience with single-dose treatment, the investigators shared their protocol with two other sites in a "multicenter trial." Again, the efficacy of single-dose amoxicillin therapy for non-antibody-coated bacterial infections was demonstrated. And again, one-third of patients were found to have antibody-coated bacteria. However, there was a marked difference in the rates of fluorescing bacteria among the three institutions. One of the new sites, Parkland Memorial Hospital, had a frequency of just over 60 percent; the other new site, Kaiser-Permanente Health Program in Oregon, showed a rate of only 8 percent. That is a big difference. It suggests that different populations were being selected for study. A fascinating final bit of information the authors glean from this multicenter effort is that antibody coating appears to be related to the duration of a woman's symptoms. The average length of symptoms prior to therapy was almost 6 days for women with antibody-coated bacteria, compared with 2 days for those in whom the assay was negative. Women in the prepaid health plan (Kaiser-Permanente) are middle-class, have easy access to the medical system, come in for care early, show a low rate of antibody coating, and respond well to single-dose therapy. Patients at Parkland are "of low socioeconomic means, without easy access to medical care, coming to the emergency ward of a municipal hospital." They have been sick longer, come to treatment with a much higher proportion of recalcitrant organisms, and are much less suitable candidates for single-dose treatment. Does single-dose amoxicillin effectively treat urinary tract infections? It depends on the patient population.

When investigators from Boston wished to test aspirin as a primary preventative for myocardial infarction, they elected to use a special group of subjects: physicians. Doctors, they reasoned, make excellent subjects in several respects.[7,8] Physicians are well informed about the risks and benefits of such a trial, they are accurate personal historians, and they are easier to track for follow-up than many people in the general population. The down side is that doctors are hardly a representative slice of America. In the Physicians' Health Study (PHS),* subjects were all male, relatively young (40 percent less than 50 years old), and had better health habits than the majority of Americans. To obtain a final study population of 22,000, over 260,000 individuals were initially invited to participate in the trial.[9] A "run in" phase was also conducted in which subjects were given aspirin for a period of 1 to 6 months. The purpose was to identify subjects who tolerated aspirin and complied with the trial design. All this enhances the internal validity of the trial considerably. We have maximized the likelihood that people will take their pills and cooperate with follow up. But it is a highly selective process. One must wonder to whom the eventual results may be generalized. Will findings apply to women, to men of less socioeconomic privilege, to those who take only two-thirds of their pills?

It is not uncommon for modern clinical trials to be confronted with this selection dilemma. If the study population is carefully screened to exclude individuals who may suffer side effects, may not comply with treatment, or have illnesses or take medications that might alter risks or commingle therapeutic effects, evaluation of the intervention is much tidier. Results are untrammeled by real-world confusions. But unfortunately, many patients do have several health problems, take a variety of medications, or occasionally forget to take the pills that give them heartburn. The most elegant trials are often conducted on a subgroup of only 10 percent of eligible subjects. No matter how convincing these findings (internal validity), one must ask, "How about the 90 percent? Would they benefit?"

Trials that are long on exclusions and high on internal validity are

---

*The Physicians' Health Study was actually designed to test *two* interventions simultaneously, aspirin for heart attack and beta carotene for cancer. Because the interventions were aimed at two unrelated health problems and the mechanisms of effect are presumed to operate independently, a "factorial design" was employed. Subjects were allocated first to treatment with aspirin or placebo then to beta carotene or placebo. Some folks get aspirin and beta carotene, some get only one of the two, and some have only placebo tablets in their pill packets. It is an efficient way to answer two questions for the price of one.

often called *explanatory trials*. Their goal is to optimize conditions for testing the intervention. Does the drug or technique work in the ideal situation? If it does not, one need bother no further. If it does, then the questions of application to the real world must be considered. A *management trial* evaluates an intervention under actual practice conditions. These two types of trials have also been tagged with the unfortunate labels of *efficacy* (explanatory) and *efficiency* (management), usages that are unfamiliar to the folks at Webster's and Funk & Wagnalls's. Because the terms are easily confused, the explanatory and management designations are preferred.

Entry criteria

Having assessed the source and general makeup of the study population, our next question should be, "Is the diagnosis accurate?" Do the people whom the investigator wishes to treat really manifest obesity, high blood pressure, or nonspecific vaginitis? Could you recognize a patient who qualifies for the intervention under discussion? How pedestrian! Of course the patient must have the illness to be included. That is only common sense. But it is dismaying to realize how often the report of a study fails to define clearly the criteria used for subject selection. The clinician must be able to identify and classify patients in the same manner as the experimenter. It is the same song of generalizability sung earlier, but it remains vital. If the investigator's definition of the problem varies markedly from your own or is unclear, you may be unable to utilize the new diet therapy, hypertension-reducing relaxation technique, or vaginal cream. You need to know whether hypertension was defined using the fourth or fifth Korotkov sound and how many readings were taken before the diagnosis was made, or whether vaginitis was diagnosed from symptoms alone, from microscopic examination of discharge, or by using cultures.

The internal validity of a trial can also be influenced by failure to adhere to clearly defined and appropriate entry criteria. Suppose a new antiarrhythmic drug has just come on the market. For want of a better name, we will call it *Nofib*. Some colleagues have tested the drug against a placebo in 100 patients admitted to the coronary-care unit for myocardial infarction (MI). The goal of their experiment is to see whether Nofib protects against sudden death. We have been asked to review the results of their experiment. "The data," they sigh, "do not look encouraging." As you see them depicted in Table 5-2, you are inclined to agree. Of the 50 patients who received Nofib, 6 died, as against 10 deaths in the comparison group. This difference, while favoring the experimental medication, is only eight percentage points and, according to a statistician hired for the occasion, is not statistically significant. It appears that the investigators have come up empty-handed.

Could problems at the point of entry have contributed to this disappointing result?

"How," we ask, "were patients selected for the study?"

"Chosen randomly from all patients admitted to the coronary-care unit with suspected myocardial infarction," comes the reply.

"What were the entry criteria?"

"The attending physician's impression of a probable heart attack."

"What cardiographic, radiologic, and serum enzyme evidence was used in determining the diagnosis?"

"It varied, depending on each admitting physician's clinical judgment."

Unfortunately, much as we revere the clinical judgment of our colleagues, general impressions and ever-present gut feelings are not acceptable entry criteria for a study. Many more people are admitted to coronary-care units for suspected or possible heart attacks than actually sustain infarctions. At least in the short term, the prognosis for persons not infarcting is more favorable than for those who have an MI. If a substantial number of entrants into the study are misclassified as having had heart attacks, the beneficial effects of Nofib may be substantially diluted. Comparison of Tables 5-2 and 5-3 illustrates how inadequate diagnosis might influence the results.

· **TABLE 5-2** ·

Effects of Nofib on survival of patients with myocardial infarction[a] ($n = 100$)

	Nofib,%	Control,%
Survived	44	40
Died	6(12)	10(20)
Total	50	50

[a]As diagnosed by physician impression.

| • TABLE 5-3 • |||
| Effects of Nofib on survival of patients with myocardial infarction[a] ($n = 50$) |||
	Nofib,%	Control,%
Survived	19	15
Died	_6(24)_	_10(40)_
Total	25	25

[a]Redefined by symptoms, ECG, and serum-enzyme criteria.

On the basis of the original data (Table 5-2), only 8 of every 100 patients (20 percent minus 12 percent) would be expected to benefit from treatment. Suppose, however, that 50 percent of the patients entered into the study were incorrectly classified. Let us also assume that survival for the patients who did not have an MI is good and that mortality occurred only among patients who really sustained heart attacks. When misclassified subjects are removed from the pool, the results appear quite different (Table 5-3). The death rate among patients given Nofib has risen to 24 percent, but the corresponding rate for patients given placebo is 40 percent. The difference in survivorship has doubled to 16 percent. Although it is possible that this difference is due to chance rather than to Nofib (as we will discuss in Chap. 8), misclassification has caused an underestimate of success.

Methods of classification

Criteria for entry into the study must be clearly stated and must constitute an acceptable definition of the disease. Methods used to classify people must also be reasonable. A problem occurs whenever sophisticated technical equipment or laboratory procedures that are not available to most practitioners are required to identify subjects who will benefit from therapy.

The work on single-dose antibiotic treatment of urinary tract infections is a case in point. The antibody-coated bacterial assay used for the studies is not a simple procedure. Urine specimens must be centrifuged and the resulting sediments washed twice in buffered saline. Washed sediments are then treated with fluorescein (conjugated antihuman globulin), incubated for 30 min, and then rewashed twice. Smears are prepared from this mixture and examined under a microscope that is specially equipped to detect fluorescence. Not exactly the kind of test available to every home and office do-it-yourselfer. Since we have already decided that we want to administer single-dose treatment only to women who do not have fluorescent bacteria (lower-tract disease), we have reached an impasse. In populations where the frequency of antibody-coated infections is high, we must be willing to risk initiating inadequate treatment of a substantial portion of our patients, or we must continue to employ conventional therapy. Fancy technology has done us in.

A similar problem occurred in a British trial evaluating therapy for hemorrhoids.[10] In this study, the authors compared a number of treatments such as anal dilatation, sphincterotomy, rubber-band ligation, and high-fiber diet. However, before patients were assigned to the different therapies, they were divided into two groups: those having "high maximal resting anal pressure" and those having "low maximal resting anal pressure." This elegant classification was determined by a means of a water-filled balloon probe and manometer. Again, we have a bit of technology that is outside the experience of most clinicians; and, as with the antibody-coated bacteria, the success of the treatment offered to hemorrhoid sufferers turns out to depend on correctly classifying them—in this instance as high- or low-pressure patients.

For clinicians who lack water-filled balloon probes, these authors offer some assistance—clinical guidelines that help distinguish high-pressure from low-pressure hemorrhoids. The high-pressure group is characterized as "young people, usually men, whose principal symptom is bleeding and anal discomfort." "Older patients, usually women, in whom prolapse is the principal complaint" usually have low anal pressures. This information is helpful and is a feature that should be sought by readers evaluating clinical trials. When a special laboratory test or technological instrument is used to classify patients and this classification is important to results, the author must provide *practical* guidelines for making this same distinction. Investigators who are mindful of the clinician's need to function with materials that are readily at hand will supply reproducible suggestions for classifying patients.

In the report of a study evaluating treatments of nonspecific vaginitis, investigators used special culture techniques for isolating the bacterium that is presumed to be responsible for the disease.[11] Very few physicians' offices or hospital laboratories would possess the capabilities for growing and identifying this organism. Furthermore, waiting for the culture to grow and for biochemical tests necessary for proper identification to be performed would take days and waste therapeutic time. These authors save the day by offering several reproducible alternatives to classifying patients with bacterial vaginitis. First, they give a detailed description of the appearance, odor, and characteristics of the bacteria-induced discharge. Then they provide a miniexperiment within the study to show that a microscopic examination of discharge to detect clue cells provides a good proxy for cultures.

To assess the problem of subject selection, ask the following as you sort through the methodology of the controlled trial:

1. Where does the study population come from? Are patients referred to specialty centers or are they typical of primary-care patients? Do they represent a spectrum of disease or a selected slice of the range of a given illness?

2. Are criteria for entry spelled out? Do the patients under study all have the disease they are supposed to have and are the author's definitions of that disease reasonable?

3. Are the techniques used for classifying subjects practical and reproducible? If methods are used that are beyond the reach of most clinicians, are suitable proxy measures offered?

CONTROLS: THEIR PRESENCE AND COMPARABILITY

Though it seems condescending to mention it, a glance to make sure that a controlled trial contains a concurrent control group is always worthwhile. Most studies nowadays evaluate a control or comparison group at the same time that they test their subjects. Comparison subjects may be given placebos, alternate treatments, or nothing at all. When authors decide that the success of their experiment will be so

• TABLE 5-4 •
Responses to placebo therapy

Condition	Number of patients	Percent relieved
Postoperative wound pain	453	31
Cough	45	40
Drug-induced mood changes	50	30
Common cold	158	35
Headache	199	52
Seasickness	33	58
Anxiety and tension	31	30
Pain from angina pectoris	122	36
Average		35

Source: Modified from Beecher.[12]

obvious that a comparison group is unnecessary, watch out! The suggestive power of thinking that you are receiving a medical treatment or innovative educational program is enormous.

Almost 40 years ago, Beecher presented a review of 15 studies that demonstrated beneficial responses to placebo therapy.[12] He showed not only a surprising magnitude of effect but also a broad range of conditions for which placebo responses could be shown. Table 5-4 illustrates some of these.

An example of the placebo effect is demonstrated in two papers that assess treatment of diabetic neuropathy with the drug phenytoin. One article reported a highly successful experiment utilizing this commonly used anticonvulsant to relieve pain among diabetics suffering from peripheral nerve problems.[13] The results were exciting! The investigator reported that 68 percent of the patients showed excellent symptomatic relief, with a "fair response" in another 17 percent. Appealing as these results appear, a red flag should flutter at the realization that the study is totally without a comparison group. When the experiment was repeated some years later,[14] investigators not only included a control group that received a placebo capsule but alternated, or crossed over, the subjects. This means that the same patients received alternating courses of the active drug, phenytoin, and the placebo and charted their symptoms without knowing which preparation they were taking.* Under the pressure of this carefully constructed experiment, the benefits of phenytoin collapsed.

A group of respected surgeons reported successful treatment of duodenal ulcer after patients swallowed a balloon which was then positioned in the stomach and continually irrigated with coolant.[15] The technique, known as gastric freezing, produced impressive results in several series of patients. Hospitals rushed to buy the hypothermia machines used to effect these cures. When controlled trials of gastric freezing were reported, the efficacy of the technique came into question. Results of a large cooperative study from five medical schools showed no benefit from gastric freezing, leaving the procedure in disrepute and many medical centers with some obsolete technology.[16]

A twist on the suggestion theme is seen in a recent study evaluating the adverse effects of the artificial sweetener aspartame.[17] In response to reports that numbers of consumers were experiencing neurological symptoms, particularly headaches, after downing diet cola or pouring packets of sugar substitute into their coffee, North Carolina investigators designed an elegant experiment to test the untoward (rather than beneficial) effects of the compound. Forty subjects who had histories of headache or related neurological symptoms that occurred shortly after consuming products containing aspartame made up the study sample. Following a thorough battery of physical and laboratory examinations, including allergy testing, subjects were administered capsules containing either measured amounts of aspartame or placebo. After a brief *washout* period that allowed subjects to rid their bodies of the chemicals, a *crossover* occurred. Those originally given the active ingredient were given placebo, and vice versa. Subjects maintained records of the adverse symptoms they experienced after ingesting the capsules and reported these to the research staff. The results are summarized in Table 5-5.

A striking similarity in the frequency of symptoms may be seen for both groups. If anything, more complaints were registered following the administration of placebo. The reason why these study subjects experienced such high reaction rates is uncertain,[17] but a

---

*Crossing patients over is a technique that is used commonly in drug trials. It has the advantages of (1) reducing the number of subjects required, since each subject serves as both an experimental subject and a control, and (2) lessening the biological variability inherent in comparing different subjects by comparing each subject with himself or herself.

• TABLE 5-5 •

**Numbers of subjects experiencing adverse effects
from aspartame or placebo**

Symptom	Aspartame	Placebo	Both treatments	Neither treatment
Headache	8	12	6	14
Dizziness	3	3	1	33
Nausea	4	5	0	31
Other symptoms	8	12	6	14

SOURCE: Adapted from Shiffman et al.[17]

certain conclusion from this study is that a good comparison group is essential.

The presence of just any comparison group is not sufficient. Ideally, controls should be selected from the same patient population as subjects who receive the intervention. Controls taken from a different patient population or chosen from an earlier period of time may not be suitable.

Consider a study that evaluated two estrogen preparations as postcoital contraceptives.[18] The study took place at five different centers, including student health services and affiliates of Planned Parenthood programs. Some 1300 women who came seeking contraception after unprotected intercourse were given one of two estrogen preparations. In analyzing the efficacy of this after-the-fact contraception, the authors compared the two different estrogens and found a small difference in pregnancy rates. No problems in this comparison. However, in an attempt to judge the overall effectiveness of postcoital contraception, they skate onto some thinner ice. Since no untreated control group was included in the original design, they compared pregnancy rates of women given estrogens with "expected pregnancy rates for one unprotected act of intercourse." These estimates are derived from other studies and turn out to be about 7/100 or 7 percent: substantially higher than the rate of only 1 percent determined for women who get the morning-after treatment. The question is whether the expected fertility rates of comparison subjects are the same as those of women coming to student health services for postcoital contraception. Chances are they are not. Estimates of pregnancy risk for the postcoital study group are based on reports supplied by the woman about her last menstrual period, when she had intercourse, and the assumption that most women ovulate 14 days prior to the onset of their menstrual period. One comparison study bases the risk of conception on data from 241 couples of "proven fertility who were experienced in using the basal body temperature method for regulating their fertility"; another comparison study group comprised married women with "presumed normal reproductive capacity" who were part of a program in artificial insemination. Now it might seem that a group of married women who are trying hard to get pregnant and carefully monitoring their ovulatory cycles would be quite different from a group of anxious young women who are seeking redress from a misadventure. These kinds of differences make it difficult to make meaningful comparisons.

The authors of the study recognized that their source populations were different, so they demonstrated that for three different populations used as comparisons, pregnancy rates were remarkably similar. This gives us at least a suggestion that their estimate of natural fertility rates may be valid. It does not, however, allay our concern that, with the anxiety and recall problems of the student health service patients, expected fertility rates for this subgroup may be considerably less than 7 percent even before postcoital contraception.

A common method of "control" is to compare results from experimental subjects with outcomes from patients treated before the new intervention was available. These are *historic controls*, and the experimental design is sometimes referred to as a *before-and-after study*. The technique has problems, as early chapters of the diethylstilbestrol (DES) story illustrate. The reason this drug, which was later found responsible for producing vaginal cancer in female offspring, was given to pregnant women in the first place was to prevent recurrent abortion. The practice proliferated after reports of dramatically improved outcomes for DES-treated pregnancies compared with outcomes for prior pregnancies.[19] Table 5-6 shows these results.

Promising as the findings appear, the value of DES did not hold up. Dieckmann et al[20] criticized the earlier work for "lack of adequate control." They suggested that patients receiving the trial medication also received more meticulous medical care and attention than they had with previous pregnancies. Factors other than DES may have been responsible for the improved outcomes. When these authors compared outcomes of pregnant women given diethylstilbestrol with those of women treated simultaneously whose management was similar in

• TABLE 5-6 •
Pregnancy outcomes of women with habitual abortion after treatment with diethylstilbestrol (DES)

	Patients	Pregnancies	Living infants	Success rate,%
Prior pregnancies	38	174	15	8.5
Study pregnancy	38	42	19	45.2

SOURCE: Modified from Davis and Fugo.[19]

every way except that a placebo pill was given in place of the active hormone, the benefits of DES vanished. Not only did DES cause serious latent side effects, but it was not effective in treating habitual abortion.

There are, unfortunately, many examples where evidence suggesting effective treatment on the basis of experiments using historic comparisons has not been confirmed when simultaneous controls were used. Sacks, Chalmers, and Smith[21] describe six such therapies, including DES.

Another variation on the comparability-of-control-group theme is illustrated in a study that evaluates the benefits of an exercise program in reducing mortality among patients who have suffered heart attacks.[22] In this study, 68 male volunteers under 51 years of age who had sustained an MI at least 5 months earlier were enrolled in an exercise program. Controls were selected from medical records of patients diagnosed as having had a heart attack who would have been eligible for entry into the program but who "for a variety of reasons did not join." The investigators came up with "matched controls" who were similar in age and number of previous infarctions to the exercise group. Results, as shown in Table 5-7, were quite impressive. The exercised patients had substantially fewer recurrent MIs and only half as many cardiac deaths as the control group.

Unfortunately, the adequacy of this control group is suspect. Why did these men who were eligible for the exercise program not participate? Reading back, we find that reasons included "family physician disapproval, shift work, lack of interest, or simply unawareness that such a program existed." Careful! One must strongly suspect that patients with a lack of interest are a very different breed from their exercising contemporaries. The authors themselves recognize

	Nonfatal recurrence	Cardiac death
• **TABLE 5-7** •		
Recurrence and death from myocardial infarction in exercise subjects ($n = 66$) and controls ($n = 117$).		
Exercise subjects	2 (3 %)	5 (8%)
Controls	13 (11%)	24 (19%)

SOURCE: Modified from Rechnitzer et al.[22]

this potential shortcoming and suggest that "subjects who enter a rehabilitation program voluntarily may differ psychologically from those who do not in a way that might affect prognosis" and that, "subjects who enter rehabilitation program frequently stop smoking and lose weight." The reduced morbidity and mortality seen in the exercisers may be due not to the experimental program but to other disparities between the compared groups that are risk factors for heart disease.

Subjects used as comparisons in controlled trials should come from the same population and be studied at the same time as subjects receiving the intervention. If there are likely to be differences in the groups under study, authors should make an effort to alert us to that possibility and provide what evidence they can muster to support similarity. Usually there is some demographic information available on subjects with which to do this. Many articles will provide a table or list comparing features like age, sex, parity, education, and so on, so readers may judge for themselves how similar the groups appear to be. Even then comparability among trial groups is not guaranteed.

THE INTERVENTION OR TREATMENT

Having scrutinized characteristics of the patients under study, let us turn our attention to the treatment or intervention itself. Therapies being offered should be carefully defined, be reproducible, and make practical sense. As we have seen before, principles that may seem self-evident are frequently ignored.

Practicality

The clinician always has the right to ask, "Is the treatment under consideration practical?" Sometimes the academicians who test these things become so involved in the intricacies of their business that they forget about some real-world constraints. When a group of investigators created an experiment to test a method for preventing travelers' diarrhea,[23] it looked as if they had come on a good thing. By giving bismuth subsalicylate prophylactically to a group of students on a tour in Mexico, the authors were able to demonstrate a 60 percent reduction in the occurrence of "tourista." Since bismuth subsalicylate comes in several well-tolerated over-the-counter preparations, it looked as if these results had much to offer to voyagers of the world. Alas, a small hitch! The medication tested comes as a suspension, and the dosage evaluated was 2 ounces taken four times each day. To achieve the desired prophylactic effect, it was calculated that a tourist traveling abroad for 3 weeks would need to carry a total supply of 168 oz, or 21 bottles, of the medication.[24] The total weight of this precautionary medication amounts to over 20 lb, leaving the traveler with a very heavy suitcase.

In fact, because the prophylactic regimen suffered from the millstone of inconvenience, duPont et al.[25] repeated their experiment using bismuth subsalicylate tablets. Employing the same setting and student population, they substituted 262-mg tablets for the bulky bottles. The tablets also proved effective at preventing diarrhea. Only 7 percent of those taking two tablets four times daily became ill, compared with 40 percent of placebo recipients. Comparable protection with much lighter luggage.

Bias

A most intriguing problem with treatments offered in controlled trials relates to compliance bias. Feinstein[26] has written about this subject and offers a number of subtle variations on the theme. Compliance bias can operate when dissimilarities in the treatments being compared create differing rates of patient adherence to the methods. If one of the therapies is a diet that is particularly difficult to follow or a medicine that tastes dreadful, study results may suggest lack of efficacy when, in fact, the explanation for the poor result is that patients failed to follow the therapy.

A good case for compliance bias can be made in the study evaluating alternative treatments for hemorrhoids.[10] Recall that in the study several surgical procedures were compared with a high-fiber diet as approaches to this troublesome condition. Diet therapy fared poorly in the comparisons, as Table 5-8 illustrates. At a 12-month follow-up, 74 percent of high-pressure patients who underwent anal dilation were improved, compared with only 27 percent of diet subjects; among low-pressure patients, rubber-band ligation gave 82 percent of subjects relief, with only 28 percent of dieters reporting success. It is possible, however, that the results reflect a compliance bias. Surgery has an aura of purposeful completion about it. We have reason to expect that the surgical procedures were carried out as advertised. Patients allocated to the diet group, on the other hand, were simply given a "high-roughage diet instruction sheet and a one-month supply of bran tablets." No fanfare and no follow-up to see how well they adhered to the diet. From what we know of medical compliance problems in general and

• TABLE 5-8 •

Clinical results 12 months after treatment of hemorrhoids by surgical procedures and diet

	High-pressure group ($n=108$)			Low-pressure group ($n=108$)		
	Anal dilation ($n=37$)	Sphincter-otomy ($n=34$)	Diet ($n=37$)	Rubber-band ligation ($n=35$)	Cryo-surgery ($n=36$)	Diet ($n=37$)
Asymptomatic	11	6	5	16	4	4
Improved	14	6	5	7	10	5
No better	5	12	13	3	7	10
Required other treatment	4	9	14	2	11	13
No follow-up data available	3	1	0	7	4	5

SOURCE: Modified from Keighley et al.[10]

unattractive diets in particular, it is reasonable to suspect that a number of patients failed to follow the plan.

The study on treatment of nonspecific vaginitis offers another example where differential rates of compliance may create a bias.[11] Among the therapies offered to women with vaginitis were a sulfonamide cream that was to be inserted vaginally twice daily for 10 days and a pill to be taken twice a day for 7 days. Use of the cream is a messy business and proper application is difficult. When the results of this study indicate the failure of the cream compared with the pills, one must wonder whether the ineffectiveness of the cream is not partly due to compliance problems.

Poor compliance can also obscure results of a clinical trial when the treatments under study have similar rates of adherence. If overall rates of compliance are low for all methods under scrutiny, beneficial effects of any of the agents may be masked. Treatment of high blood pressure has always been plagued by compliance problems; people just will not take their pills. Suppose we were trying to compare a new antihypertensive agent with one of the standard treatments available. Both medications are tablets that are taken twice daily. Neither medication has an offensive taste or intolerable side effects. In other words, we anticipate no difference in compliance. However, it turns out that the patients we are studying are very relaxed about taking their prescribed medications. When it comes time to look at the results, we find little improvement in the control of high blood pressure among patients taking the new agent compared with those on the old therapy. However, we also discover that only 20 percent of patients took their pills regularly. Under these circumstances, it is very difficult to know whether or not the drug under study has a beneficial effect. As in the Nofib example where medication effects were diluted by including improperly diagnosed heart-attack patients, low overall compliance may hide a real benefit.

Of course, the compliance issue can be viewed from another perspective. While one may argue that an unpalatable diet or noxious medicine cannot be dismissed as ineffective until we have assured ourselves that noncompliance has been controlled, noncompliance is a reality. It exists as a practical impediment in day-to-day medical care. The clinical trial that includes noncompliers may give a more accurate picture of the value of an intervention in the real world. Patients are going to have difficulty using vaginal cream properly, following rigorous diets, or lugging 20 lb of Pepto-Bismol to Mexico. Authors who acknowledge and analyze potential compliance problems are more help to the clinician than those who simply exclude nonadherent patients from consideration or take heroic steps to make sure that patients follow instructions.

Competing interventions

While we are contemplating the treatments used by investigators, we should consider the possibility that cointerventions are occurring. A cointervention, as the names implies, is another, usually unrecognized, form of treatment that is taking place at the same time as the intervention under study. A cointervention may play a major role in achieving the results but receives no credit. To bias results of the study, cointerventions must not only be responsible for the effects observed but be unevenly distributed between treatment groups. Suppose we were looking for evidence that anticoagulants given to patients recuperating from myocardial infarction prevented thromboembolic disease and reduced mortality. Patients with heart attacks are assigned to two different units within the hospital. In one they receive anticoagulants therapy and in the other none. We find at the conclusion of our trial that there were significantly fewer deaths among patients in the anticoagulation group. But just as we are about to sound the fanfare and publish our results, we discover that patients admitted to the unit that was administering anticoagulants also received prophylactic antiarrhythmic agents and had early ambulation. These are cointerventions that may boast partial or total responsibility for the improved mortality seen in our experimental unit.

Cointerventions may be a factor in the trial evaluating the therapies for hemorrhoids.[10] Patients receiving surgical procedures, for example, may be given adjunct treatments that affect their outcome. Postoperative patients are commonly prescribed topical ointments, sitz baths, and pharmacological stool softeners; often, they are encouraged to use bran and high-roughage diets. The use of any of these additional treatments would render interpretation even more difficult.

In some intervention studies, particularly those in which a subject's behavior is the target of treatment, the risk to validity is not that intervention subjects do not comply with treatment but that control subjects do. If members of the comparison group change their habits in a manner that lowers risk for the outcome of concern, apparent benefits of intervention may be diminished or even lost. Perhaps the best-known example comes from the large multiple-risk factor intervention trial known as MRFIT.[27] This ambitious project evaluated the effects of reducing high blood pressure, elevated cholesterol, and cigarette smoking on rates of cardiovascular disease. Over 12,000 men who were determined to be at high risk from some combination of these risk factors were assigned to either a "special intervention" or a "usual care" group. Special-intervention subjects had diet counseling to lower their cholesterol, were placed in smoking cessation programs, and underwent medical protocols to reduce their elevated blood pressures. Usual-care subjects were referred back to their regular health providers.

Subjects in both groups were followed for an average of 7 years. At completion of the trial, rates of death from coronary heart disease, cardiovascular disease, and all causes were compared. Heart disease and cardiovascular deaths were reduced among special-intervention subjects by 7.1 and 4.7 percent, respectively, a slight and not statistically significant improvement. The overall death rate of the special-intervention group was actually a few percentage points higher—rather disappointing results after 10 years of effort!

Investigators offered several interpretations of these findings. The first, of course, was the possibility that the intervention simply had no effect on mortality. But a second possibility was that the benefits may have been masked by an unanticipated improvement in the risk profiles of the usual-care subjects. Indeed, the control subjects had, as a group, lowered their blood pressures, reduced their smoking, and dropped their cholesterol levels over the course of the trial. While their improvements were not as great as those in the special-intervention group, the risk reduction may have been sufficient to obscure the benefits of the interventions. The fact that death rates for both groups were substantially lower than had been predicted at the start of the trial lends support to this theory. Based on best estimates available in 1972, when the trial began, investigators anticipated a coronary heart disease death rate of 29 per 1000. In fact, mortality from coronary heart disease was 18 per 1000 in the special-intervention group and 19 per 1000 among the usual-care subjects.

A number of characteristics of the intervention, then, must be carefully considered:

1. Is it clearly defined so as to be reproducible in other settings? Are dosages and details of techniques stated and consistent with current practices?

2. Are the methods under examination practical? Could treatments be used in a variety of medical settings or are they suitable only for the fantasy world of academics?

3. Is there a potential for compliance bias? Are the treatments under study sufficiently different in application that differential rates of adherence are likely? If so, has the author addressed this issue and attempted to assess actual compliance for the interventions?

4. Are competing interventions occurring? If so, are they unequally distributed among treatment groups? Has the author looked for these and tried to assess their potential impact?

ALLOCATION: SUBJECT ASSIGNMENT

Subjects must be allocated by the investigators. This is the activity that gives the controlled trial its special shine, but it also offers yet another opportunity for biases to slip in to tarnish the results. While many people speak of the "randomized controlled trial" as if this term were all one word, *random allocation* of subjects is only one technique in use. As the term *random* gets tossed about rather casually, it is worth reminding ourselves precisely what it means. Randomly assigning subjects does not mean that the investigator grabs everyone sitting on the north side of the waiting room and plops them into group A, leaving folks sitting on the south side to form group B. The goal of proper subject allocation is to avoid selection bias that might create unwanted differences in comparative groups. People might congregate on the north side of the waiting room because the chairs are softer there and easier on their arthritic joints or because their friends from work sit there. Systematic differences between these people and their counterparts on the other side of the waiting room might affect results of the study. The problem is cut of the same cloth as the convenience sampling discussed in Chap. 4. Convenience allocation opens the way to bias. While it may be done with best intentions of being unselective, problems can occur.

Random allocation, on the other hand, is a very carefully planned method of assigning subjects that avoids bias. It may be accomplished by making assignments from a table of random numbers, using calculator programs that generate random numbers, or even drawing numbers from a hat; but for true random assignment to take place, each subject must have an equal chance of being assigned to any of the study groups at hand. Only by using this rigorous method of allocation can we guard against the unconscious biases of the assigning investigators and, indeed, the study subjects themselves.

An example of biased allocation comes from a study that attempted to assess the risks and benefits of delivering babies in a special birthing room.[28] In this experiment, a group of 500 women was offered the chance to deliver in a "bedroom type room next to the delivery suite." Amenities included a queen-sized bed, casual furnishings, and a large private bathroom. Also included in the birthing-room delivery plan was a series of agreements between patients and staff which included avoidance of intravenous fluids, fetal monitors, excessive analgesia, and much of the paraphernalia associated with traditional in-hospital deliveries. The patients participating in this birthing-room experience were compared with a "similar number of low-risk mothers and babies in the standard delivery room." The results of the study suggest not only that the birthing room was safe but also that deliveries occurring there had fewer complications for mother and baby than deliveries under standard conditions. The author evaluated 42 perinatal outcomes in the two groups and found that birthing-room deliveries had a significantly lower rate for 12 complications, including cesarean sections, fetal distress, jaundice, congenital anomalies, and child abuse.

The author registers happy surprise at what he terms the "unexpected" results; but the reduced rate of complications in the experimental group is probably not unexpected. Let us review exactly how subjects were allocated to the birthing room and standard-care groups. Participants in the birthing-room deliveries were volunteers. They were assessed for risk factors and only low-risk subjects remained eligible for the study. Factors placing women into the standard-care group are not clearly specified except that these women were also said to be low-risk.

Are the groups comparable? Are the so-called risk factors that may influence the outcome of pregnancy equivalent in both? We know that the patients differ in one important respect: one group volunteered to participate in the birthing-room experiment while the other women did not wish to partake. Could this difference affect results? We are supplied with little information about characteristics of these two groups of women that might help us decide. However, we know enough about volunteers in health programs to make a guess that the birthing-room volunteers were probably somewhat older, better educated, and of higher socioeconomic status and parity than the comparison women. Since these factors are known to be associated with a favorable outcome of pregnancy, we again have a situation where the intervention, the birthing room, appears to produce lower complication rates when, in fact, improved outcomes are a manifestation of allocating a healthier group of women to the experimental group. Women interested in birthing rooms are likely to produce bigger, bouncier babies regardless of the type of delivery employed.

Had the author of this study randomly allocated only subjects who were willing to undergo the birthing-room experience, patient-selection biases might have been avoided and the results been very different. An elegance of allocation is illustrated in a Canadian study on a similar subject.[29] Investigators in this report wished to explore the possible benefits of the Leboyer approach to childbirth, a method that promotes birth in a dark, quiet room, delayed clamping of the umbilical cord, and calming of the infant by massage and bathing in warm water. To guard against lack of comparability between the Leboyer and "conventional delivery" groups, all subjects, before they were entered in the study, were required to fulfill eligibility requirements that included a low obstetrical risk score and interest in the Leboyer approach to childbirth. Random assignment was then made, so that each woman had an equal chance of being delivered by the Leboyer or the conventional method. As things turned out, the authors were unable to demonstrate any important advantage to soft lights and tepid baths when compared with a conventional albeit gentle delivery.

Even allocation methods that would appear to be free from bias can present problems. Gifford and Feinstein describe a fascinating example in discussing experiments evaluating the use of anticoagulants for myocardial infarction (MI).[30] In a study performed in the late 1940s, patients admitted to hospital with the diagnosis of acute

MI were placed on anticoagulants or left untreated, depending on the day of the week. On odd days, patients received anticoagulants; on even days they served as controls. Although this system of allocation would seem to be a vast improvement over that described for the birthing-room experience, questions of bias were raised. Physicians who were admitting patients to these hospitals were aware of the nature of the study that was being conducted. They knew that if the date was even, their patients would go untreated. Such knowledge might sit poorly with a doctor who had already concluded that anticoagulants were beneficial. If it were the waning hours of June 16 and he had a patient in the emergency room who had chest pain but was not severely ill, the temptation would be great to let the hour of midnight slip by before admitting the patient to the ward. A slight delay in the emergency room could assure the patient of receiving the anticoagulant therapy.

How could this bias results? The outcome being evaluated in this experiment was mortality, and there are many factors other than anticoagulants that may affect a patient's survival following a heart attack. Among the best predictors of outcome are the severity of the heart attack and the patient's condition at the time of admission to hospital. The only patients for whom physicians could reasonably delay admission to gain access to the anticoagulant dates would be patients with less severe illness. Patients in shock or with arrhythmias would not be good candidates for this bit of strategy; nor would they be good candidates for survival. So if a number of patients who were less ill and had a more favorable prognosis were systematically included in the anticoagulation group, survival would appear spuriously high and anticoagulants would garner undeserved praise for prolonging life. An intricate bit of business, but it may well have happened.

Even strict randomization in a clinical trial can fall prey to unexpected events. Investigators in another trial looking at anticoagulants and heart attack felt they were protecting themselves from bias by randomly assigning patients to receive heparin or serve as controls by a system of sealed envelopes.[31] To their dismay, they discovered that anticoagulant anarchists were having their way again and were trans-illuminating the envelopes to foil the random allocation.

Stratification The foibles of human nature notwithstanding, random allocation is the method of choice for controlled trials. But even when this is executed properly, there is a risk that randomization will not accomplish its intended purpose. Random assignment attempts to equalize experimental and comparison groups by giving each subject an equal chance to be in any of the groups; but chance is chancy business, as anyone who has flipped coins or played cards can avow. Just as it is possible to come up with heads for 8 out of 10 flips of the coin, so can groups assigned by the random process turn out to be dissimilar in their makeup.

The investigators who assessed the effect of exercise on recurrent MI recognized that allocation problems might have played mischief with their earlier endeavor.[32] So when they undertook a large randomized trial with over 700 participants to test the role of high-intensity exercise compared with light exercise on the prevention of recurrent MI, they took no chances. Even though subjects were assigned to treatment categories by unbiased random allocation, the researchers checked to see if, in fact, their two study groups turned out to be comparable. Table 5-9 shows how closely both groups compare for a variety of known cardiovascular risk factors. Similar

· TABLE 5-9 ·		
Characteristics of subjects at entry to high- and low-intensity exercise interventions		
Characteristic	High-intensity exercise ($n=379$)	Low-intensity exercise ($n=354$)
Median age	47.3	47.7
Previous infarcts (%)		
0	91.6	90.7
1	6.6	7.3
2	0.5	0.3
3	0.3	0.6
Hypertension (%)	17.7	14.7
Blue-collar occupation(%)	42.2	41.0
Type A personality (%)	69.9	71.2
Current smoker (%)	34.6	36.4
Cholesterol (median, mg/100mL)	217	216

SOURCE: Adapted from Rechnitzer et al.[32]

tables help readers gauge the success of allocations by how closely intervention and comparison groups are matched.

Bias can occur any time groups being compared are unequal with respect to either risk factors that predispose to disease or existing conditions that may influence outcome. While there are methods for dealing with unanticipated inequalities when data are analyzed, most investigators would rather not be victimized by the noncomparability problem in the first place. If important risk factors or comorbid conditions (concurrent illnesses that may influence outcome) can be identified at the outset, subjects may be grouped or prognostically stratified prior to assignment. Feinstein has written extensively about prognostic stratification and its importance in interpreting clinical trials.[26]

In the Leboyer childbirth example, the investigators were savvy enough to use prognostic stratification to avoid the pitfalls of this multirisk situation. Before assignment, patients were grouped according to parity and social class, and random allocation proceeded separately within each subgroup. The likelihood that high-risk first pregnancies will end up being compared with less risky subsequent pregnancies because of chance maldistribution is thus minimized.

Prognostic stratification was also used by Rechnitzer et al. in their Exercise-Heart Study and is one reason their study groups enjoyed similar risk profiles.[32] Subjects were stratified by variables such as hypertension, presence or absence of angina, type A behavior, and employment status prior to allocation. Alas, after all this marvelous methodological care was taken, the high-intensity exercise program showed no advantage over light exercise in the prevention of recurrent heart attack.

ATTRITION

As with observational follow-up studies, subjects who drop out of a clinical trial present problems. Not only are their data lost but the nagging question arises whether attrition is related to treatment and could affect outcome. If so, the stage is set for biased results. A large multicenter Norwegian study assessed the benefits of timolol, a beta-adrenergic blocker, on reducing mortality among patients recovering from myocardial infarction.[33] Patients were randomly assigned to receive timolol or a look-alike placebo and were monitored for up to

36 months. Not surprisingly, some patients dropped out of the study. The attrition rate was significantly higher among patients receiving timolol than among those receiving placebo and was most pronounced during the first month of the study. The authors analyzed reasons for participant withdrawal and discovered that timolol patients withdrew most frequently because of symptoms of hypotension and bradycardia, well-known side effects of the drug. This differential dropout rate presents an analysis problem. Once patients are no longer taking the drug, they are no longer receiving the benefits of beta blockade and should not be considered when the drug's effectiveness is assessed. On the other hand, patients who withdraw because of timolol's side effects may have labile cardiovascular physiology, making them susceptible to sudden death. If this high-risk group of patients were excluded, timolol might appear effective not because its pharmacologic action prevented cardiac events but because its side effects forced susceptible subjects out of the study.

To meet this challenge, the authors invoked a principle known as *analysis by intention to treat*. They looked at their data in two ways, both excluding and including dropouts in the analysis. The study design defines deaths occurring during or within 28 days of the end of treatment as outcome events. When data were viewed this way and dropouts were excluded, there were 67 deaths among timolol-treated patients compared with 117 deaths among a similar number of placebo-treated patients. When deaths were evaluated according to the original treatment assignment, by intention to treat, and dropouts were included even though they did not receive a full course of drug, the differential between timolol and placebo was little changed: 98 and 152 deaths, respectively. By either method of analysis, the benefit of timolol was demonstrated and the question of attrition bias satisfactorily resolved.

These two methods of analysis do not always produce such harmonious results. Sackett and Gent[34] discuss the results of a study comparing surgical and nonsurgical treatment of transient ischemic attacks (TIAs) among patients with bilateral carotid artery stenosis. When treatment success was based on follow-up of patients who had been discharged alive and free of stroke after hospitalization, surgical treatment appeared to be superior. It provided a 27 percent reduction in recurrent TIA, stroke, or death. However, a number of patients entered into the study did not qualify for follow-up. Of the original 167 patients entered in the trial, 16 died or had strokes while in the hospital. Only 1 of these was medically treated, and 15 had surgery. When data from these patients were included in the analysis, the risk reduction from surgery fell to 16 percent and no longer appeared significant. Sackett and Gent discuss guidelines for helping readers cope with these differing results.[34]

END POINTS

Readers should give some thought to the "end points" or outcomes that are reported in clinical trials. The usual caveats apply. Are the effects of the intervention clearly defined? Are they comparably determined? Do the end points selected include the most important possible outcomes of the trial? Several trials that have shown promise in reducing mortality from a specific cause have been disappointing when deaths from other causes were considered. In the Physicians' Health Study,[35] a 44 percent reduction in heart attack was found for physicians who took low-dose aspirin. This salutary news was dampened by a trend toward increased hemorrhagic stroke among treated subjects and an undiminished overall death rate from cardiovascular causes. How does one interpret such results? The aspirin appears to be performing its role of platelet inhibition quite well. But if no overall reduction in deaths can be detected, is the trial a success?

Consider which end points are meaningful. When a Utah law was passed requiring training of individuals who serve alcohol in restaurants and bars to provide "more responsible beverage service," an experiment was conducted to assess the effects of the intervention.[36] In all, 97 servers and 43 managers, representing 26 establishments, took part in a 1-day training session. For comparison, 14 establishments of similar size and type where training had not yet occurred were selected. Participants completed pre- and postsession questionnaires that measured their beliefs and knowledge about responsible alcohol service. One month following the education program, trained observers visited the establishments to observe actual practice.

The pencil-and-paper results were encouraging. Servers and managers demonstrated better knowledge and attitudes about responsible serving practices. Unfortunately, behavior did not follow suit. No differences were noted between intervention and control establishments in the ways in which servers communicated with customers or limited the delivery of drinks.

It is also important to consider *when* an end point or outcome occurs in relation to the intervention. There is a window of time during which it is reasonable to assume that arrhythmias are affected by beta blockers or lung cancer rates are influenced by smoking cessation campaigns. Outcomes that occur long after subjects stop taking a drug or before benefits of an intervention can logically be expected can complicate the analysis. There are "gray zones" where proper attribution becomes difficult.

SUMMARY

This all seems like a tremendous amount of effort to expend just looking at the methods of controlled trials, but by now certain of these principles should have a familiar ring. The problems of comparability of comparison subjects and the forces of selection that go into choosing exposed or experimental subjects have come up before in discussing case-control and follow-up designs. The principles are the same. The reader has a right to expect an author to supply the information necessary to generalize from the specific study to other populations. We can likewise expect that care has been used in selecting comparison subjects, and that when questions of comparability arise, the author will provide information about how subjects and their controls are similar and how they differ.

Although experimental designs, like follow-up studies, are not encumbered by recall bias and problems encountered in using data from the past, they share the plague of attrition. Both of these prospective designs depend upon following subjects over time to assess outcomes. The risk that patients will drop out of the project because they are depressed or are unable to comply with a complicated diet is a constant threat to results.

Comfort in assessing these methodological pitfalls comes only with practice—reading lots of studies and scouring the methodology for problems. But remember, flaw catching can become a disheartening addiction, since very few studies are free of blemish. If you look hard enough, weakness may be found in the most robust of designs. We must guard against dismissing a study because of defects that are relatively unimportant. When flaws are found, we must ask whether the problems will impinge upon the validity of the study. In cases such as the birthing-room experiment, where great potential for bias exists from the unequal distribution of risk factors in the two groups, the problem is crippling. After assessing this design, one would do well to proceed to other reading tasks. In other cases, such as the case-control study of sudden infant death syndrome, recall bias, though a potential threat, probably did not have a major impact on results.

Investigators, like the rest of us, are subject to the imperfections of humanity. They concoct and serve up their studies with the best of intentions. Often the seasoning is not quite right and sometimes critical ingredients are missing or misapportioned. Have compassion for the cooks; try to distinguish between small matters of taste and major indigestibilities.

REFERENCES

1. Hill AB: *Principles of Medical Statistics*, 9th ed. New York, Oxford University Press, 1971.
2. Sackett DL: Design, measurement and analysis in clinical trials, in Hirsch J, Cade JF, Gallus AS, et al (eds): *Platelets, Drugs and Thrombosis*. Basel, Karger, 1975.
3. Louis TA, Shapiro SH: Critical issues in the conduct and interpretation of clinical trials. *Ann Rev Public Health* 4:25, 1983.
4. Chalmers TC, Smith H Jr, Blackburn B, et al: A method for assessing the quality of a randomized control trial. *Controlled Clin Trials* 2:31, 1981.
5. Fang LST, Tolkoff-Rubin NE, Rubin RH: Efficacy of single-dose and conventional amoxicillin therapy in urinary-tract infection localized by the antibody-coated bacteria technique. *N Engl J Med* 298:413, 1978.
6. Rubin RH, Fang LST, Jones SR et al: Single-dose amoxicillin therapy for urinary tract infection: Multicenter trial using antibody-coated bacteria localization technique. *JAMA* 244:561, 1980.
7. Hennekens CH, Eberlein K: A randomized trial of aspirin and beta-carotene among U.S. physicians. *Preventive Medicine* 14:165, 1985.

8. Hennekens CH: Issues in the design and conduct of clinical trials. *JNCI* 73:1473, 1984.
9. Steering Committee of the Physicians' Health Study Research Group: Preliminary report: findings from the aspirin component of the ongoing physicians' health study. *N Engl J Med* 318:262, 1988.
10. Keighley MRB, Buchmann P, Minervini S, et al: Prospective trials of minor surgical procedures and high-fibre diet for haemorrhoids. *Br Med J* 2:967, 1979.
11. Pheifer TA, Forsyth PS, Durfee MA et al: Nonspecific vaginitis: Role of *Haemophilus vaginalis* and treatment with metronidazole. *N Engl J Med* 298:1429, 1978.
12. Beecher HK: The powerful placebo. *JAMA* 159:1602, 1955.
13. Ellenberg M: Treatment of diabetic neuropathy with diphenylhydantoin. *NY State J Med* 68:2653, 1968.
14. Saudek CD, Werns S, Reidenberg MM: Phenytoin in the treatment of diabetic symmetrical polyneuropathy. *Clin Pharm Ther* 22:196, 1977.
15. Wangensteen OH, Peter ET, Nicoloff DM et al: Achieving "physiologic gastrectomy" by gastric freezing. *JAMA* 180:439, 1962.
16. Miao LL: Gastric freezing: An example of the evaluation of medical therapy by randomized clinical trials, in Bunker JP, Barnes BA, Mosteller F (eds): *Costs, risks, and benefits of surgery.* New York, Oxford University Press, 1977, pp 198-211.
17. Schiffman SS, Buckley CE, Sampson HA et al: Aspartame and susceptibility to headache. *N Engl J Med* 317:1181, 1987.
18. Dixon GW, Schlesselman JJ, Ory HW, Blye RP: Ethinyl estradiol and conjugated estrogens as postcoital contraceptives. *JAMA* 244:1336, 1980.
19. Davis ME, Fugo NW: Early pregnancy complications. *JAMA* 142:778, 1950.
20. Dieckmann WJ, Davis ME, Rynkiewicz LM, Pottinger RE: Does the administration of diethylstilbestrol during pregnancy have therapeutic value? *Am J Obstet Gynecol* 66:1062, 1953.
21. Sacks H, Chalmers TC, Smith H Jr: Randomized versus historical controls for clinical trials. *Am J Med* 72:233, 1982.
22. Rechnitzer PA, Pickard HA, Paivio AU et al: Long-term follow-up study of survival and recurrence rates following myocardial infarction in exercising and control subjects. *Circulation* 45:853, 1972.
23. Dupont HL, Sullivan P, Evans DG et al: Prevention of traveler's diarrhea (emporiatic enteritis): Prophylactic administration of subsalicylate bismuth. *JAMA* 243:237, 1980.
24. Gorbach SL: How to avoid running with *Escherichia coli. JAMA* 243:260, 1980.
25. DuPont HL, Ericsson CD, Johnson PC et al: Prevention of travelers'

diarrhea by the tablet formulation of bismuth subsalicylate. *JAMA* 257:1347, 1987.

26. Feinstein AR: *Clinical Biostatistics*. St Louis, Mosby, 1977.
27. Multiple Risk Factor Intervention Trial Research Group: Multiple risk factor intervention trial: Risk factor changes and mortality results. *JAMA* 248:1465, 1982.
28. Goodlin RC: Low-risk obstetric care for low-risk mothers. *Lancet* 1:1017, 1980.
29. Nelson NM, Enkin MW, Saigal S, et al: A randomized clinical trial of the Leboyer approach to childbirth. *N Engl J Med* 302:655, 1980.
30. Gifford RH, Feinstein AR: A critique of methodology in studies of anticoagulant therapy for acute myocardial infarction. *N Engl J Med* 280:351, 1969.
31. Carleton RA, Sanders CA, Burack WR: Heparin administration after acute myocardial infarction. *N Engl J Med* 263:1002, 1960.
32. Rechnitzer PA, Cunningham DA, Andrew GM et al: Relation of exercise to the recurrence rate of myocardial infarction in men: Ontario exercise-heart collaborative study. *Am J Cardiol* 51:65, 1983.
33. The Norwegian Multicenter Study Group: Timolol-induced reduction in mortality and reinfarction in patients surviving acute myocardial infarction. *N Engl J Med* 304:801, 1981.
34. Sackett DL, Gent M: Controversy in counting and attributing events in clinical trials. *N Engl J Med* 301:1410, 1979.
35. Steering Committee of the Physicians' Health Study Research Group: Final report on the aspirin component of the ongoing physicians' health study. *N Engl J Med* 321:129, 1989.
36. Howard-Pitney B, Johnson MD, Altman DG et al: Responsible alcohol service: A study of server, manager, and environmental impact. *Am J Public Health* 81:197, 1991.

CHAPTER SIX

MAKING MEASUREMENTS

I am giddy; expectation whirls me round.

TROILUS AND CRESSIDA, Act III, Scene II

$\mathcal{W}$e have ruminated over study designs; tasted some problems, such as selective recall, loss to follow-up, and compliance bias; and sampled several solutions, such as matching, stratification, and random allocation. We are ready now to consider the implementation of these designs—that is, to examine how measurements are made and data acquired. After struggling with the complexities of study methodologies, gathering data would seem a straightforward proposition. By now it should come as no surprise that there are problems in this domain as well.

When measurements are made and data are collected, errors can occur. Children are improperly measured or their heights are incorrectly plotted on the growth curve; a centrifuged hematocrit tube is not correctly read; items on a personality-inventory scale are inadvertently left blank or filled in incorrectly. The list of unfortunate possibilities is almost endless, and the chance that data acquired by researchers do not properly measure the attributes they wish to determine is a potent hazard. Although errors in data collection can occur anywhere in the process—from obtaining measurements on a patient through keying in data for computer analysis—we will focus on problems that occur at the interface between patients and investigators. It is here that the most serious errors occur and the only point at which readers have a shot at detecting difficulties. We will discuss two general types of errors, those that occur in an unpredictable fashion and those that are made in a biased, systematic way.

RELIABILITY AND VALIDITY

Two terms that readers will encounter whenever measurements are mentioned are *validity* and *reliability*. We have already discussed the concept of validity as it applies to the overall acceptance of study results (whether conclusions are justified based on design and interpretation) or in the case of external validity (whether results can be generalized to settings and subjects outside those described in the study). As used to describe data, validity refers to the degree to which a measurement represents a true value, such as how closely a blood-pressure determination represents a patient's true blood pressure or a hematocrit estimates the actual packed cell volume. Reliability relates to the reproducibility of measurements. How closely do repeated measurements on the same subject agree? Both these attributes are important to clinical studies and are related. Errors can be caused by a lack of either validity or reliability. If six student nurses attempt to measure a patient's blood pressure and obtain values that range from 110/70 to 145/95 mmHg, the results lack reliability. This creative group of estimates may be due to changes in the patient's anxiety level, differences in inflation of the cuff, or variable auditory acuity among the students. The results also lack validity. Better reproducibility is necessary to achieve a valid result but does not guarantee it. If a cuff of the wrong size is employed or the manometer is out of calibration, each of our six nurses might come up with a blood pressure reading of 145/95 mmHg, a totally reliable finding that does not represent the true pressure.

VARIABILITY OF THE
UNSYSTEMATIC SORT

Over the past 30 to 40 years we have come to appreciate an amazing spectrum of variability that occurs when health researchers or health providers attempt to make clinical measurements. Problems of reliability pervade every aspect of clinical work, from history taking and the physical examination to laboratory and x-ray investigations. In part, the problem is due to subject variation. Pulse rates and blood pressures may change from one observation to the next. A patient who swears to the medical student that he is a teetotaler may admit to taking the occasional beer when questioned by the attending physician. Human frailties on the part of observers also contribute. Examiners become fatigued, are inattentive, or simply have not been trained to make measurements in a standardized manner. Regardless of the underlying reason, observers assessing the same subject, the same symptom, the same skin rash, or the same blood smear frequently come up with differing interpretations.

In a study by Derryberry on "the reliability of medical judgments on malnutrition,"[1] six pediatricians were asked to independently examine 108 eleven-year-old boys and rate their nutritional status. Each boy was examined by each physician and rated on a four-point scale that ranged from "excellent" to "poor." In the author's understated prose, "the results of this investigation were disconcerting." Ratings of the six physicians showed marked variation. One physician rated 15 of the 108 boys as having poor nutritional status, another rated only 2 in that category. Twenty-five different boys were given the "poor" rating by at least one of the doctors, and only one child received a unanimous judgment of poor by the entire group of evaluators. Two youngsters received every rating from excellent through poor in the course of the six evaluations.

Even elements of the physical examination that would pretend to high objectivity are subject to observer variability. Meade et al. report on differences among three physicians of "comparable clinical experience" who were given the task of palpating the peripheral pulses of 84 hospitalized patients.[2] For this experiment, the examiners had only to record whether a particular pulse was present or absent. To spice up the game, 12 of the patients were recycled through the examination so that they were evaluated twice by each of the three observers. Table

6-1 summarizes some of the findings from this study. Agreement ranged from as high as 97 percent for palpation of femoral pulses to as low as 69 percent for the dorsalis pedis pulse. If this interobserver problem were not bad enough, the 12 patients who underwent a second pulse check highlighted further deficiencies. Intraobserver error—that is, a rater's change from a previous assessment—also occurred. When the three examiners were checked on the 48 pulses that they assessed on two occasions, they changed their minds about the presence or absence of a pulse from 13 to 27 percent of the time.

The pronouncements of those who interpret the technological trappings of medicine are not immune from the problems of observer variation. Lack of agreement among experts reading coronary angiograms,[3] electrocardiograms,[4] and radiographs[5] has been demonstrated. In 1947, a group of investigators wished to compare the effectiveness of four different radiographic techniques for use in tuberculosis case-finding programs.[5] Their strategy was simply to take radiographs of the same patients using the different methods and have the films interpreted by a group of experts—in this case, five members of the Veterans Administration Board of Roentgenology. While the investigators suspected that differences in interpretation would occur in the course of the study, they were surprised by the magnitude of the variability problem. For 1200 radiographs that were read independently by each of the five observers, the number of interpretations that were positive for tuberculosis ranged from 56 to 100. Again, there was no uniform agreement as to which these cases were, with 131 different films interpreted as positive by one or more of the readers. Intraobserver problems were also demonstrated as films were reread and observers changed their interpretations from previous readings.

· TABLE 6-1 ·

Agreement of three observers examining femoral, posterior tibial, and dorsalis pedis pulses in 96 male patients (192 observations)

	Agreement, all present	Disagreement, present/absent	Agreement, all absent	Percent total agreement
Femoral	187	5	0	97
Posterior tibial	126	40	26	79
Dorsalis pedis	105	59	28	69

SOURCE: Adapted from Meade et al.[2]

As it all turned out, observer consistency proved to be such a problem that the comparison of the four radiologic techniques became a secondary issue. The variability of observers posed a greater limitation to accurate diagnosis than the radiographic method utilized.

Even assessments we revere as "gold standards" are susceptible. In an exercise related to a multicenter trial exploring the effects of beta carotene on cervical dysplasia, four pathologists were asked to examine and grade 106 biopsy specimens.[6] Each slide was reviewed by each pathologist, who rated the specimens as belonging in one of five categories of dysplasia: (1) none, (2) mild, (3) moderate, (4) severe, and (5) carcinoma in situ (CIS). Variability for the readings of the 106 slides may be seen in Table 6-2.

The table shows the percentage of agreement when the first pathologist's readings are compared to those of the other three pathologists. The italicized numbers (running diagonally) represent complete agreement, with cells furthest from the diagonal representing the greatest discord—a bit of tarnish to be sure.

The catalog of observer problems should strike a concordant note with clinicians. Everyone experiences measurement disagreements, as any medical student can attest after having failed to palpate the 2-cm liver edge or hear the systolic heart murmur that the senior resident or attending physician uncovered. We should realize, however, that experience does not grant immunity from the problem. In the exam-

• **TABLE 6-2** •

Percentage agreement of four pathologists' classification of cervical dysplasia on 106 slides (comparison with "index" pathologist)

Grade of dysplasia, "index" pathologist	Grade of dysplasia, three pathologists				
	None	Mild	Moderate	Severe	CIS[a]
None	*35*	47	12	6	0
Mild	7	*54*	30	8	1
Moderate	1	21	*50*	26	2
Severe	1	7	35	*49*	8
CIS	0	6	19	54	*22*

[a]CIS = carcinoma in situ.

SOURCE: Adapted from DeVet et al.[6]

ples we have just discussed, the variant observers were often experts in their fields. They have as much trouble as the rest of us.

Most of the errors we have been discussing occur in a haphazard or unpredictable fashion. They can be a nuisance, since without reasonable measurement reliability, the validity of study results will be compromised. However, minor, random variations tend to even out—some higher and some lower—and, human imperfectibility being what it is, can never be entirely eliminated.

SYSTEMATIC ERROR

There are, however, more dangerous brands of error. These occur when variations in measurements take on a predictable or biased aspect. An example comes from a study devised to determine the accuracy of clinical measurements of fetal heart rates.[7] In this investigation, an electronic monitor was attached to record the intrauterine heart rate. At the same time, members of the hospital staff counted the heartbeats by auscultation. Observer variations in the range of 20 percent of the monitored rate were discovered. However, the pattern of this variability did not occur randomly. Fetal heart rate is a guide to the infant's well being. A rate in the neighborhood of 130 to 150 beats per min suggests that labor is progressing satisfactorily. Heart rates that fall below 130 or rise above 150 suggest that problems may be brewing and that the fetus is experiencing distress. Figure 6-1 depicts the patterns of observer variation that occurred with different monitored fetal heart rates. When the true rate is within the 130-to-150 range, observer errors appear evenly scattered between overestimates and underestimates; but if monitored rates rise or fall to levels that indicate distress, the pattern of errors no longer appears symmetrically distributed. When the monitored rate drops below 130, observer errors tend to overestimate the rate, that is, bring it back toward the desirable range. When the rate exceeds 150, there is a tendency for observers to make estimates on the lower side of the electronic value.

This represents biased error. The cause for the bias is understandable; the hospital staff is not looking for trouble. The staff wants healthy deliveries and babies with good outcomes. Nevertheless, the message is clear. As with poor, giddy Troilus, expectation plays tricks

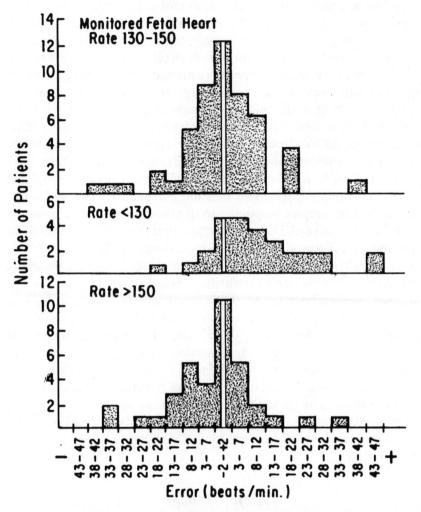

FIGURE 6-1 Error of auscultation of hospital staff at different fetal heart rates. (From Day et al.[7] Reprinted by permission.)

on the mind. The wishes of the observer can influence measurements. Opportunities for measurement bias are abundant in medical studies and are one more problem that journal readers need to sniff out.

Investigator and interviewer biases

Measurement biases can be produced on both sides of the investigator/subject dyad. For those who are collecting information for a study,

the pitfalls are numerous. One's investment in the results or anticipation of how subjects are likely to respond can easily become a self-ful-
filling prophecy. This is not to impugn the integrity of investigators.
Objectivity is difficult to master. It is difficult for surgeons not to find
benefits from their favorite operative procedures to alleviate hemorrhoids or for social workers—looking for evidence of abuse and
neglect—not to uncover child maltreatment in a group known to be
at high risk. It is unfair to expect an investigator trying a new antihypertensive agent to display total disinterest when taking the blood
pressure of a subject under treatment. Even when investigators are
not directly involved in data gathering, difficulties can occur. Choi and
Comstock evaluated the effect that the personalities of hired interviewers had on subject responses to questionnaires in a community
mental-health survey.[8] The instrument, administered by six different
interviewers, measured a variety of mental-health characteristics, including sensitive items like troubles with alcohol, suicidal thoughts,
nervous breakdowns, and stressful life events. In checking for observer
variation, the authors noted that interviewer C produced subject
scores that differed substantially from those of her colleagues. When
the investigators attempted to identify items in the questionnaire that
interviewers found embarrassing, interviewer C reported feeling un-
comfortable with questions pertaining to suicide, menstruation, marital happiness, and personal habits; none of the other five interviewers
seemed disturbed by these topics. The authors concluded that a measurement bias was operating—that the personality and beliefs of the
particular interviewer were systematically affecting responses on her
questionnaires.

Subject biases

Subjects can also introduce bias into the data-collection process. When
subjects are invested in the experiment, have ideas about which
therapy might be preferred, or simply want to please investigators by
responding in a favorable way, results may be altered. Patients who
believe that a certain method of childbirth is beneficial are likely to
report high satisfaction and favorable outcomes for their infants;
parents of hyperactive children who have become convinced that food
additives cause their child's aberrant behavior will see improvement
in symptoms when these toxins are eliminated from the diet. Most
patients want things to be better. They want to do things right! In fact,

there is such a tendency for subjects to wish to respond in what they perceive as a correct fashion that the term *social desirability bias* has been coined to describe the phenomenon.

This bias has been demonstrated in evaluations of health-education programs designed to encourage the use of car seats for young children. Pediatricians and other health professionals would love to find better ways of assuring the safe transport of infants and toddlers. Studies have evaluated a number of parent-education techniques, including cautionary displays and pamphlets in the doctor's waiting room, staff demonstrations of the proper use of car seats, and counseling by physicians themselves on the proper use of auto safety equipment. The success of the strategies, however, depends more on how measurements are made than on the educational method employed.

Two studies conducted on military populations acquired data in different ways and came up with disarmingly different results. In the first study, parents of infants visiting a pediatric practice for a 4-week checkup were allocated to receive one of four health-education strategies.[9] At the 8-week follow-up visit, these parents were questioned regarding their use of car seats. As can be seen from Table 6-3, a small but tangible increase in proper restraint use appeared for families who received the health-education message from nurses or doctors. The evidence for this success, however, came from parents' self-reports. Having been instructed by the practice to use car seats, parents were then quizzed about how well they obeyed instructions. This is fertile ground for producing a social desirability response bias.

• TABLE 6-3 •

Reported use of acceptable restraints for infants aged 8 weeks in passenger automobiles after various parent-education strategies

Education strategy (100 in each group)	Unsatisfactory restraint	Satisfactory restraint
None	91	9
Display	88	12
Pamphlet	92	8
Nurse	78	22
Physician	78	22

SOURCE: Modified from Scherz.[9]

When another army officer looked at the same health-promotion problem, he assessed it in a different fashion.[10] Access to his base was limited through two gates, both guarded by members of the military police. He had the MPs record the restraint status of all children in automobiles passing through the gates. Then, for 18 months, he diligently attempted to educate parents during well-baby visits and prenatal classes. The rate of car-seat use among children failed to improve when habits were again observed by the MPs. At the same time, parents "almost uniformly stated in the pediatric clinic that they [had] and [used] a safety seat."

Another source of consternation for investigators trying to observe subjects and collect data on them is the fact that the act of observation may change the behavior. This phenomenon goes under the fancy name of the *Hawthorne effect* (named not for a person but for a manufacturing plant where the effect was observed). The essence of the problem is that people may act differently when they know they are being watched. Examples of particular interest to clinicians come from projects that attempt to alter physician behavior, such as studies that try to improve the way doctors order laboratory tests or prescribe medications. Generally these efforts aim at educating physicians and stressing logical approaches to better decision making. Beneficial effects demonstrated in these experiments may as often be due to the Hawthorne effect as to planned edification, however. Evidence to support this suspicion is found in the typical pattern that physician behavior follows in the wake of interventions. Inappropriate test ordering or prescribing generally decreases for a time, creating a satisfaction in the investigators that comes from watching rational enlightenment. Delight is usually short-lived, however. Given a few additional months, behavior reverts to its previous wayward level, suggesting that the transient improvement was related to the presence of the study rather than its message.

The report of an evaluation of an educational program to reduce ordering of thyroid function panels demonstrates this rebound phenomenon.[11] Here the authors attempted to influence physicians' laboratory utilization during an educational conference in which doctors could characterize and analyze their motives for test ordering. In the 3-month period following the conference, the ordering of thyroid panels dropped (see Fig. 6-2). However, as time went on and clinicians forgot either what they had learned or about the dark shadow of the

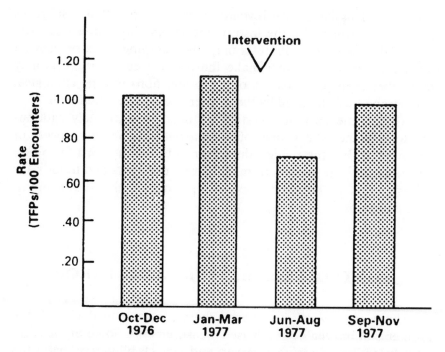

FIGURE 6-2 Rate of ordering thyroid function panels (TFPs) by 3-month quarters. (From Rhyne and Gehlbach.[11] Reprinted by permission of Appleton and Lange.)

investigators hovering over their shoulders, rates returned toward preintervention levels.

In the course of studies on practitioner/patient interactions, Starfield and colleagues found evidence that presence of an observer in the room with the doctor and patient changes the practitioner's recognition of patient problems.[12] When medical records completed after visits that were observed were compared with those of visits where no observer was present, it was found that a significantly higher percentage of patients' previous concerns were noted when the observer was in attendance.

Increasing comfort or familiarity with the measuring devices used to collect data may also affect subject response. It has been noted, for example, that patients having their blood pressures measured for the first time are much more likely to have elevated readings than after they have become acclimated to the medical setting. Studies that utilize pretests and posttests to measure knowledge or repeat administrations of psychological inventories run the risk that a subject's earlier experience with the instrument will modify scores of subsequent administrations. Pretests may give learning clues or provide test-taking experience that make the posttest easier; subjects may remember their previous responses to questions in a psychological battery and be influenced by these when they are retested later.

All this means that investigators must be extremely cautious not to influence the course of human behavior in the process of observing it. For the reader, the lesson is to be on guard for biases introduced by the process of making measurements and to look for evidence that authors have taken steps to minimize the errors of data collection.

CONTROLLING MEASUREMENT ERROR

There are several steps researchers can take to deal with the problems of unreliable and biased measurements. Some of them are already familiar. Keeping observers and subjects blind is probably the best known technique for reducing bias. In the *double-blind* trial, neither the investigator nor the subject is allowed to become aware of which particular intervention is being used for any given subject. This approach is particularly suited for drug trials, where identical pink capsules can be concocted to contain the placebo and the active drug. There are some obvious limitations. It is very difficult, for example, to conceal the queen-sized bed and rococo decor of a birthing room from either physicians or patients. When measurements are made on interventions where investigators cannot maintain ignorance of the allocation, independent observers from outside should be brought in. In the Leboyer childbirth study described in Chap. 5, for example, outcome assessments of neonates were made by observers who were kept scrupulously unaware of the method of childbirth used to bring the baby into the world.[13]

There are other techniques for improving measurement reliability and minimizing observer error. These include the following:

Establishing unambiguous standards When all observers are clear on exactly how measurements are to be made, variability is reduced. Agreement on what size blood-pressure cuff should be used for which size arm and whether the fourth or fifth Korotkov sound should be used as the diastolic estimate will produce more reliable blood-pressure measurements. Deciding in advance how many millimeters an ST segment must be elevated to be compatible with an infarction pattern on an electrocardiogram will improve the consistency of the diagnosis of heart attack. Measurement devices should, of course, be standardized and calibrated.

Providing observers with supervised training and practice Once the guidelines for measurements have been established, observers need to practice their interviewing skills or measuring techniques to see where variations or biases are likely to occur. Training need not be extensive or elaborate to improve measurement validity. As part of a national study of the relationship of colon polyps to cancer, a proficiency testing program was begun to monitor the accuracy of interpretation of fecal occult blood tests.[14] Eight coordinators from clinical centers were tested with preprepared stool samples *before* a 1-h instructional seminar, *immediately after* the seminar, and *several months later.* Instruction focused on the proper addition of reagents and correct interpretation of color changes for the test. Findings are presented in Table 6-4.

Overall, the percentage of slides read correctly increased from 60 percent for the preintervention period to 91 percent in each of the postintervention periods. Most of this improvement was seen for the intermediate, "moderately positive" samples.

Using multiple observers or data sources Although we have recognized the problems that multiple observers have in agreeing with

• TABLE 6-4 •			
Percentage of correctly interpreted hemoccult tests before, immediately after, and several months after training			
Reading	Before	Immediately after	Months after
Strongly positive	78	97	100
Moderately positive	38	90	94
Negative	94	81	86

SOURCE: Adapted from Fleisher et al.[14]

one another, several opinions are usually better than one. It is good form, for example, when diagnostic studies such as radiographs or pathology specimens are involved in results, to send these bits of gold to independent observers for a second opinion. Even projects that rely on data acquired through seemingly straightforward methods such as chart audits are better served when information is checked by more than one observer. Use of multiple sources of data is another useful technique for improving validity. Recall from Chap. 3 that Ross et al. use medical records and pharmacy records to verify the estrogen use reported by subjects[15] and Wynder and Graham performed a special substudy to demonstrate the reported smoking habits of cases and controls were not influenced by investigator bias.[16]

Knowledgeable researchers will assess interrater reliability and supply readers with estimates of how closely different raters agree. The information is usually offered in terms of percent agreement or a *correlation coefficient*, with higher values signifying better reliability. Better still are reports that provide estimates of agreement that have taken chance into account. When the four pathologists sort cervical cytology slides into five categories,[7] chance alone dictates that there will be some concordant groupings. The study investigators report reliability as a *kappa value*, meaning that they have statistically adjusted their findings to account for this chance agreement.

While there are few guarantees that a research article is free from measurement error, readers may derive some comfort from evidence that an author has been rigorous in the pursuit of objective data. As with investigators who demonstrate cognizance of study-design problems such as attrition bias, authors who set forth the methods they use to guard against measurement error are more likely to gain our confidence.

SUMMARY

When measurements are made, errors will occur. Pay particular attention to whether authors have

1. Attempted to improve reliability by (a) establishing unambiguous measurement standards, (b) utilizing trained observers, and (c) corroborating observations with second opinions.

2. Taken steps to guard against biased measurement. Where possible, are both subjects and investigators blind to subject allocation? If the identity of treatments cannot be concealed, are attempts made to incorporate independent observers who are unaware of study hypotheses or treatment allocations?

REFERENCES

1. Derryberry M: Reliability of medical judgments on malnutrition. *Public Health Rep* 53:263, 1938.
2. Meade TW, Gardner MJ, Cannon P, Richardson PC: Observer variability in recording the peripheral pulses. *Br Heart J* 30:661, 1968.
3. Detre KM, Wright E, Murphy ML, Takaro T: Observer agreement in evaluating coronary angiograms. *Circulation* 52:979, 1975.
4. Davies LG: Observer variation in reports on electrocardiograms. *Br Heart J* 18:568, 1956.
5. Birkelo CE, Chamberlain WE, Phelps PS, et al: Tuberculosis case finding: A comparison of the effectiveness of various roentgenographic and photofluorographic methods. *JAMA* 133:359, 1947.
6. DeVet HCW, Knipschild PG, Schouten HJA, et al: Interobserver variation in histopathological grading of cervical dysplasia. *J Clin Epidemiol* 43:1395, 1990.
7. Day E, Maddern L, Wood C: Auscultation of foetal heart rate: An assessment of its error and significance. *Br Med J* 4:422, 1968.
8. Choi I, Comstock GW: Interviewer effect on responses to a questionnaire relating to mood. *Am J Epidemiol* 101:84, 1975.
9. Scherz RG: Restraint systems for the prevention of injury to children in automobile accidents. *Am J Public Health* 66:451, 1976.
10. Walsh MJ: Physician involvement in safety programs is not enough. *Pediatrics* 61:142, 1978.
11. Rhyne RL, Gehlbach SH: Effects of educational feedback strategy on physician utilization of thyroid function panels. *J Fam Pract* 8:1003, 1979.
12. Starfield B, Steinwachs D, Morris J, et al: Presence of observers at patient-practitioner interactions: Impact on coordination of care and methodologic implications. *Am J Public Health* 69:1021, 1979.
13. Nelson NM, Enkin MW, Saigal S, et al: A randomized clinical trial of the Leboyer approach to childbirth. *N Engl J Med* 302:655, 1980.
14. Fleisher M, Winawer SJ, Zaubner AG, et al: Accuracy of fecal occult blood test interpretation. *Ann Intern Med* 114:875, 1991.
15. Ross RK, Paganini-Hill A, Gerkins VR, et al: A case-control study of menopausal estrogen therapy and breast cancer. *JAMA* 243:1635, 1980.

16. Wynder EL, Graham EA: Tobacco smoking as a possible etiologic factor in bronchiogenic carcinoma: A study of six hundred and eighty-four proved cases. *JAMA* 143:329, 1950.

CHAPTER SEVEN

INTERPRETATION: DISTRIBUTIONS, AVERAGES, AND THE NORMAL

An obese statistician named Rouse
To his physician would continually grouse
"My head and feet are so little
And I bulge in the middle."
Said the doc, "You're quite 'normal,' by Gauss."

A normal, red-blooded American boy is regarded as the ideal, but weather that is normal for the time of year is just the usual. The average physician is a standard representative of the breed; an average student is a bit dull. It is normal for a 2-year-old child to engage in thumb sucking because it is typical behavior; a normal electrocardiogram means no heart disease. The average score on a biochemistry examination is the mathematical midpoint; the statistical patterns of weights and heights collected on a group of college freshmen are noted to be normal distributions. Not since Chap. 2 have we run up against such challenging semantics! But where the terminology for study designs was burdened by many terms that described a handful of concepts, we now find a variety of meanings attached to several words. The confusion arises when we begin to describe and interpret the data generated in medical studies. In this chapter we examine ways in which techniques used to summarize data get misapplied and the confused interpretation that can result.

FREQUENCY DISTRIBUTIONS

Whenever we begin accumulating data—whether blood-pressure measurements from a community screening program, the hemoglobin values of women in a prenatal clinic, or the National Board scores of third-year medical students—there is a need to organize our findings. One effective way of summarizing data is to create a frequency distribution, which is a map that depicts the number of times individual hemoglobin levels or board scores are found within the population being sampled.

Frequency distributions come in a variety of shapes and sizes. The most notorious was made famous by a gentleman named Gauss, a German mathematician who lived in the early nineteenth century. Gauss put forth the "law of errors," which states that repeated measurements made on the same physical object fall in a predictable pattern or distribution that has certain mathematical properties and predictive features. Plots of Gaussian or normal distributions form a bell-shaped curve, a lovely symmetrical affair with a rounded peak in the middle and gracefully descending sides that approach but never quite reach zero (see Fig. 7-1A). Repeated measurements of the length of a table will show slight variations about the true value; readings close to the actual length will cluster toward the middle of the distribution and occur with relatively high frequency, while larger variations from the true length will be less common and will distribute themselves toward both ends of the curve. Well enough! However, it was not long before Gauss's law had been borrowed and applied to the grouping of measurements made on *different* objects. The presumption was that if multiple measurements of a single individual's height were found to form a bell-shaped distribution, the heights of different individuals within a large group might just fall into a similar pattern. Over the years, the convenience of this assumption—that biologic variation occurs in a Gaussian or normal pattern—has swept aside the niggling warnings of purists that the assumption is incorrect. Elveback

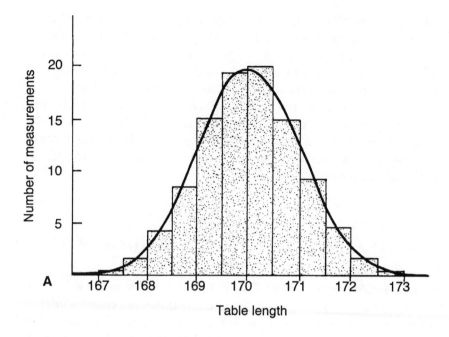

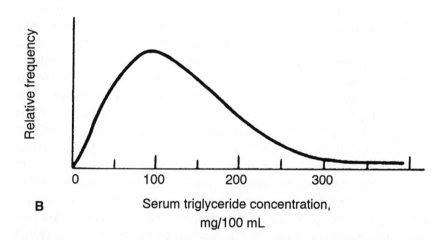

FIGURE 7-1 *A*. **Normal distribution. Repeated measurements of a table's length.** *B*. **Skewed distribution. Serum triglyceride levels.** (*B*: from Leaverton, PE: *A Review of Biostatistics: A Program for Self-Instruction,* 3rd ed. Boston, Little, Brown, 1986. Reprinted by permission. Copyright © 1986, Little, Brown and Company.)

and colleagues plotted the frequency distributions of a number of common laboratory tests and found they varied from the Gaussian mathematical approximations.[1] In general, the actual patterns of the biological measurements formed skewed distributions, meaning that the curves were asymmetrical, with one side of the curve extending out in an elongated fashion (see Fig. 7-1*B*). Despite outcries against this misappropriation of mathematical theory, the notion that the normal distribution is a good approximation of the frequency pattern of biological measurements has become entrenched in medical thinking and medical writing.

MEASURES OF CENTRAL TENDENCY

To facilitate discussion about distribution, several summary descriptors are in common use. These are the attributes of *central tendency* and *variability*. These concepts are not new to most readers, but because some misunderstandings have occurred over the years, a bit of review and clarification is worthwhile. The data in most distributions tend to cluster or center about a certain point as they array themselves along a range of possible values. By far the most commonly used measure of central tendency is the arithmetic mean, or what most people speak of as the average. The *mean* of a distribution is derived by summing the individual values and dividing by the total number of determinations in the sample. The mean is a useful measure for conveying a general idea of where a population stands with respect to a given measure. If the women in a prenatal clinic have a mean hemoglobin of 8.6 g, more concern about nutritional status might be raised than if the mean were 12.0 g. A mean score of 70 by a medical school class on the anatomy section of the National Board examinations—when the national average was 87—could prompt a detailed look at the school's curriculum. An average pulse rate of 54 beats per minute for a group of men completing a cardiac rehabilitation program suggests a conditioning effect when compared with a baseline mean pulse rate of 78. Less familiar but also useful as indicators of central tendency are the median and the mode. The *median* of a distribution is a midpoint at which one-half the observations fall below and one-half above the value. The *mode* is the most frequently encountered measurement in the distribution.

In bell-shaped Gaussian distributions, the mean, the median, and the mode all land at precisely the same location, so that any of the three descriptors offers the same view of central tendency. However, as distributions become skewed, the three characteristics can be located at different points along the curve (see Fig. 7-2), and it becomes a matter of some debate as to which most fairly represents the distribution.

As an illustration, recall the study on the natural history of bacteriuria in schoolgirls.[2] This report described the long-term follow-up of a cohort of schoolgirls who were found, during a school screening program, to have asymptomatic urinary tract infections. Figure 7-3 shows the frequency distribution of reinfections experienced by these subjects compared with the recurrence rate for the group of girls who served as controls. The distribution is markedly skewed. It shows that while most girls experienced relatively few reinfections, 20 percent had recurrences numbering 5 or more. The mean number of reinfections was between 2 and 3, but this was not the usual experience. Most girls (the mode) did not have any, and the midway point of distribution (the median), where one-half had more and one-half had less, is 1. The arithmetic mean of a distribution like this one is quite misleading.

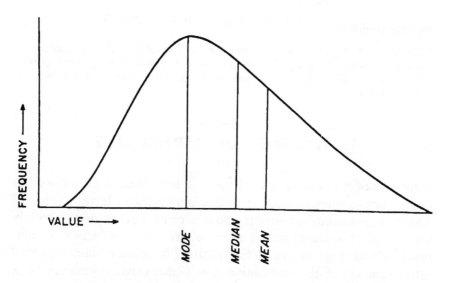

FIGURE 7-2 Variable locations of the mean, median, and mode in a skewed frequency distribution.

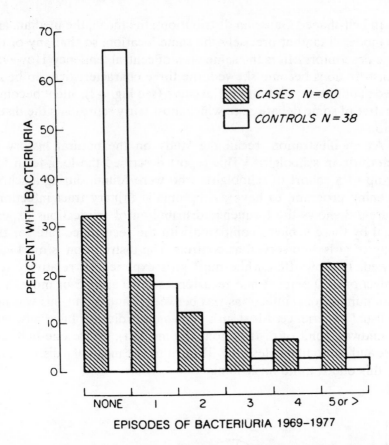

FIGURE 7-3 Episodes of bacteriuria in schoolgirls during follow-up studies of those showing the condition in screening programs. (From Gillenwater et al.[2] Reprinted by permission of the *New England Journal of Medicine*.)

INDICATORS OF VARIABILITY

Estimates of the centers of distributions do not tell us all we need to know about arrays of data. It is also important to have a sense of whether measurements group about a central point or are widely spread. Do cholesterol values or anxiety scores of our study population all cluster together, or do they scatter? If we are making repeated measurements on the same subject, as Gauss originally suggested, a distribution that hovers tightly about the mean suggests good measurement reliability. If we are measuring different individuals in a population, little variability suggests homogeneity among study subjects. Several estimators of variability are commonly employed. The *range* simply identifies extreme limits of a distribution. The weights of subjects in the experimental diet program ranged from 248 (the lowest) to 352 (the highest) pounds. Another guide to variability is the standard deviation. The *standard deviation* is calculated from a formula that sums the squares of differences between the group mean and each individual value. The greater these differences, the more spread the distribution and the larger the standard deviation. The notation commonly seen is "mean ± SD," and reference is frequently made to values that are one or two standard deviations from the mean. Within the span of one standard deviation on either side of the mean, we may expect to find approximately 68 percent of the values in a normal frequency distribution; within two standard deviations lie 95 percent of the observations, and three standard deviations on either side of the mean encompass 99 percent of the values in the distribution. Figure 7-4 depicts all this. It is a convenient way of describing variation; but, as we will see, it has been subjected to some misappropriations.

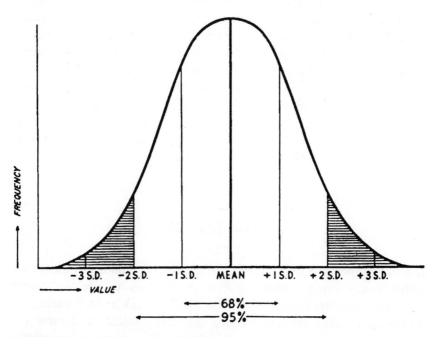

FIGURE 7-4 Areas included within 1, 2, and 3 standard deviations (SD) of the mean for normal distributions.

A third way of looking at the variations of a distribution is to use *percentiles*. Just as the median is the 50th percentile of a collection of data, the 75th or 95th percentiles can be determined and indicate that a particular head circumference or serum creatinine level lies at a point where it is larger than 75 percent or 95 percent of the other values in the group. An advantage of dividing distributions into percentiles is that it may be legitimately accomplished without respect to the shape of the distribution. Unlike the interpretation of standard deviations, the percentile system does not rely on the assumption of an underlying normal distribution.

Estimates of variability are useful descriptors. They give a perspective that means or medians alone cannot provide. Suppose you are attempting to decide on the therapeutic efficacy of cephalexin for treatment of lymphadenitis due to *Staphylococcus aureus*. You learn that the level of drug in the blood needed to eradicate all the strains of *S. aureus* that lurk in your neighborhood is about 12 μg of drug per milliliter of serum. You find a report that offers the graphic information depicted in Fig. 7-5A.[3] This chart shows the mean serum levels of cephalexin at various time intervals following administration of a standard dose of the drug. It is easy to see from the curve that the peak levels of the drug exceed the concentrations required for eradication of the bacteria. It is also easy to forget that the graph depicts only the mean or average levels achieved in the experiment. When information on the variability of drug levels is included, as in Fig. 7-5B, important information is added. With the bars depicting the range on either side of the mean, it becomes apparent that there is enough variability in absorption of the drug that the level of 12 μg will not be reached some of the time. Summarizing data by use of the mean alone without some indications of variability can be misleading.

NORMALITY

If averages are a potential point of confusion, major psychoses can result from trying to make sense of the ambiguous use of the term "normal." As suggested earlier, the word has taken on a number of meanings ranging from attributes that are typical or common to indicators of health to ideals to which we aspire. Murphy has written several papers on the subject and describes seven nuances of meaning

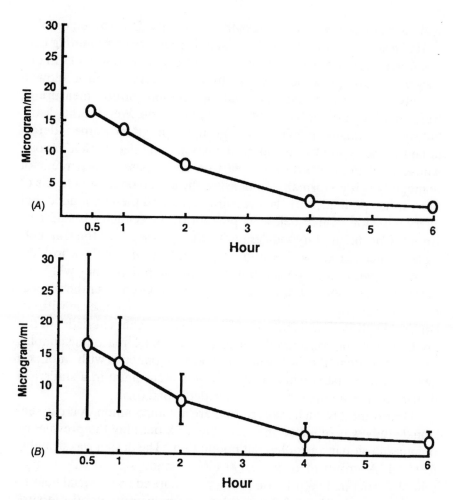

FIGURE 7-5 *A.* Mean serum levels of cephalexin following an oral dose. *B.* Mean and range of serum cephalexin levels following an oral dose (range indicated by vertical lines). (*B:* from Barton and Feigin.[3] Reprinted by permission.)

for the term.[4-6] Feinstein[7] and Sackett[8] also offer discussions on the topic. By far the biggest problem for clinicians comes from confusing the normal of statistical distributions with the presence or absence of disease. When Gauss defined his normal distribution, he certainly never dreamed that phrases like "within normal limits" and "outside of the normal range" would become standard medical jargon.

Most clinicians appreciate the fact that the boundaries of illness are not always clear, especially when we begin discussing problems such as anemia, high blood pressure, or obesity. Does a hemoglobin of 10.5 g signify ill health? Will a diastolic pressure of 90 mmHg lead to early death? Is 200 lb too much for a 6-f 1-in man to weight? In our passion to distinguish between health and disease, we have allowed ourselves to pretend that statistical distributions offer a measure of truth that they do not have the power to provide. We plot the distribution of hemoglobin values for a group of pregnant women, determine the mean and two standard deviations, and decide that anyone whose level falls outside the area that encompasses 95 percent of hemoglobins is abnormal. We measure the serum potassium levels of our cardiac patients, sort the measurements, and then announce that everyone with a value below 95 percent of the readings is suffering from the problem of hypokalemia. It is easy to see how the trap gets baited, since we know that a great percentage of people who have anemia or who develop symptoms of potassium deficiency will have hemoglobin or potassium values at the lower extremes of the respective distributions. But arbitrarily assigning subjects a disease without considering the clinical features of the disease or characteristics of the population being considered makes no sense. Such reasoning enables us to argue that the heaviest 5 percent of patients with anorexia nervosa are, in fact, overweight. To allow a cut point in a statistical distribution to define a disease is decidedly bad form.

Unfortunately, such indiscretions are not uncommon. A cross-sectional study was reported that set as its task defining the prevalence of hypertension in an adolescent population.[9] The design was straightforward. A group of over 10,000 eighth-grade students in a large school district had their blood pressures recorded by a special health-screening team. Wary of the problems of measuring blood pressure accurately, the investigators added some nice touches to minimize observer error. Members of the screening team underwent special training and were periodically monitored for reliability. Measurements were taken with a random zero mercury manometer, a device especially designed to reduce potential observer bias. Students were even allowed to sit quietly for 4 minutes before their pressures were obtained so as to minimize the effects of anxiety and activity. A very sound approach that unfortunately was not sustained.

Once all 10,000 blood pressure measures were obtained, they were arranged in a giant distribution and divided into percentiles. Then, with a pronouncement that resounds with plausibility, the authors announce that about 9 percent of the adolescents screened had either systolic, diastolic, or both systolic and diastolic pressures above the 95th percentile. The conclusion is that these children are abnormal, that they have evidence of hypertension. Surprising results? Not exactly. It is a perfect circle of reasoning. If you create distributions of measurements, divide them into percentiles, and then define as diseased the upper 5 percent of systolic pressures and the upper 5 percent of diastolic pressures, it is easy to make a pretty good guess what the prevalence of hypertension is likely to be—about 5 percent for each group. In point of fact, there is no reason to suspect that any of these children has hypertension. The 95th percentile levels for systolic and diastolic pressure found from this initial screening were about 130 and 75 mmHg, respectively. These values are well below levels of adult blood pressure that begin to correlate with the disease manifestations of hypertension. In the final analysis, none of the 10,000 subjects had a sustained diastolic pressure of 90 mmHg or more. Statistical distributions simply cannot be used to identify disease. The madness of this method is perhaps more dramatically illustrated by the use of normal distributions and standard deviations to define normal ranges of laboratory tests. Here the goal seems admirable enough—to provide clinicians with guidelines for interpreting laboratory data. Subtle mischief is afoot, however. When the clinician receives a report offering information that a patient's serum uric acid, bilirubin, or cholesterol level is outside the normal range, how does the news get processed? What does it mean? Usually physicians translate "outside normal limits" to mean "abnormal"; abnormal means "unhealthy" and unhealthy means "diseased." The syllogism is not totally unreasonable. After all, we know that people who have gout suffer from high uric acid levels, that liver disease is characterized by abnormally high bilirubin concentrations, and that increased levels of cholesterol in the blood are associated with coronary artery disease.

The question is, how closely associated with disease are these abnormal chemistries? The answer requires knowing how the laboratory folks who produce these normal limits go about their business. Just what constitutes a normal range, and what sort of population sample is used to determine normality? It is rarely evident from the laboratory reports, but typically, normal limits are concocted by the old standard-deviation routine. Uric acid or bilirubin determinations are performed on a large sample of blood specimens, a distribution is constructed, and the area that contains 95 percent of the values is blocked off to represent normality. Are values that lie outside this hallowed zone really abnormal? Do they represent disease? That depends upon who the reference subjects are. If the technicians, custodians, and administrators who work at the laboratory comprise the sample, or volunteers from the local college or nursing school, it is likely that few or none of them will have gout or obstructive liver disease. They are all healthy; yet by selecting the extremes of the distribution, 5 percent are automatically identified as abnormal or diseased. As with the adolescent hypertensives, it is an exercise in logical tail-chasing. There are also some interesting economic implications.

In an age of polylaboratory, commercial biochemical laboratories have made financial hay out of semantic confusion. By providing useful, normal values to aid interpretation of test results, they have created profit from uncertainty. If a population of healthy adults is used to determine the distribution of uric acid or cholesterol values and the two standard-deviation cutoff points are used, 5 percent of nondiseased subjects will have values categorized as abnormal. With automation, multiple determinations are possible on a single blood sample at little increase in cost over a single test. However, when 5 percent of each of 20 biochemical determinations are routinely classified as deviant, the likelihood that any nondiseased individual will have all 20 determinations reported as normal is only 36 percent. (The probability that each test will be normal is 0.95; that of test A being normal and test B being normal...and test T being normal is $0.95 \times 0.95... \times 0.95$. For 20 tests that is 0.95^{20}, or 0.36.) Clinicians who order multitest panels on patients must either ignore frequently occurring abnormal values or repeat the test in hopes that aberrant values will return to the normal range. Repeating the panels creates the potential for further classification errors and more confusion while also adding substantially to the medical bill. Sackett has discussed this problem and summarizes the situation quite nicely[8]:

> The use of a statistical concept such as the standard deviation to set the limits of normal for clinical laboratory tests represents the cross-sterilization of disciplines, for it represents taking a misunderstood concept from sampling statistical theory and misapplying it in an individual clinical situation.

A final morsel for the normal stew, entitled "Microcephaly in a Normal School Population,"[10] presents the spectrum of confusion that surrounds normality. The author of this paper sets as the major objective for his study "to examine the prevalence of microcephaly, defined as a head circumference greater or equal to two standard deviations below the mean, in a normal school population." We are off to quite a start. Microcephaly, while literally meaning the condition of having a small head, has connotations of abnormality—that is, of being associated with mental retardation. That is the only reason it is worthy of concern. The prevalence of microcephaly in a normal school population tastes of the non sequitur—"normal" in this case suggesting without disease or mental handicap.

The author gathers a group of approximately 1000 students aged 5 to 18 years who are attending regular classes in a suburban school district. Head circumferences of these youngsters are measured and compared against a standard to determine the frequency of microcephaly. Nineteen children, or 1.9 percent of the population, fall into this abnormal group. The author remarks,

> ... the finding of 1.9 percent prevalence of microcephaly in a normal school population was not unexpected, since the author anticipated that there would be a significant number of children with microcephaly and normal intelligence enrolled in regular classrooms.

He is certainly correct in his expectation. Finding a 1.9 percent prevalence of microcephaly, when microcephaly is defined as the lower 2 percent of a frequency distribution, should not be unanticipated. It is a given. Examining the reference standard used in classifying children, we find that the standard was derived in exactly the same manner as the experimental data were obtained, by measuring the head circumferences of a large number of presumably healthy children. The author reaches the dramatic conclusion that "although head-circumference measurement remains a valuable clinical tool, a head-circumference measurement greater than two standard deviations below the mean is not uniformly associated with mental retardation." We cannot help but agree with him since, as he also points out, "our population was selected from children attending regular classrooms [and] mentally retarded children with microcephaly would not be included in the study population." The study is an exercise in confused logic and imprecise usage—interchanging concepts of "usual" and "healthy" with arbitrary cut points in statistical distributions.

REGRESSION TO THE MEAN

There is one last bit of business about interpreting distributions that readers should master. It has to do with an impressive sounding phenomenon called *regression to the mean*. Regression can occur any time investigators classify subjects according to measurements that lie at the extremes of a distribution and then remeasure them. On average, the repeat values will appear less extreme; that is, they will regress toward the mean of the total population. Studies describing hypertension detection and treatment programs are at substantial risk of demonstrating this regression phenomenon. Typically, a group of shopping-center browsers submit to having their blood pressures taken. These pressure determinations form a frequency distribution with a mean of perhaps 120/80 mmHg. At the upper end of the distribution are a number of people whose diastolic pressures exceed 90 mmHg. These people are labeled hypertensive and are the individuals on whom follow-up and treatment attention will be lavished. They are offered pills, weight-control programs, relaxation training, or biofeedback, and a gratifying response is found. At follow-up, the average diastolic pressure of the group has fallen. It is concluded that therapy has been successful. While some of this improvement may be due to treatment, part of it is inevitably due to regression.

Remembering from Chap. 6 about the unavoidable variability of measurements, we should recognize that classification errors will occur in a one-shot screening attempt. Given the combined effects of the physiological variation of individual blood pressures and measurement error, misclassifications are bound to occur. If we use 90 mmHg as our dividing line for designating hypertension, there will be people whose true diastolic pressure is 89 mmHg but who measure 96 mmHg on the occasion of the screening. These people will be misclassified as hypertensive. Of course, errors in classification occur in the other direction as well; a person whose true diastolic pressure is 95 mmHg may register 88 mmHg on screening day and be relegated to the non-hypertensive group. However, when we screen and establish a cutoff, we immediately lose interest in people who fall below the 90 mmHg mark; they never get measured again and remain incorrectly grouped. We reassess only those people whose pressures are found to be high. Since some of them have been misclassified, subsequent blood pressure determinations will tend to restore them to their rightful places as nonhypertensives. The result is that, on average, the group designated as having high blood pressure will have lower pressures the second time around. Figure 7-6 is a schematic representation of the problem.

The study that screened Texas eighth-graders for high blood pressure demonstrated the regression effect quite nicely.[9] In the first round of blood pressure measuring, 9 percent of the adolescents had "high blood pressure." These young people were then reexamined on two occasions before a final figure of 1.6 percent was announced as the prevalence of hypertension. Since no treatment was involved in this program, there must be some other explanation for the "normalizing" of so many of the subjects who were classified as hypertensive initially.

In part, the reduction probably reflects decreased anxiety on the part of students as they became familiar with the measuring situation. Patients frequently display mild elevations in blood pressure on a first visit to the clinic; this disappears on subsequent visits. Regression to the mean is also operating. The key to this effect is the repeated measurement of only subjects initially classified as over the arbitrary cut point of the distribution—in this example, those with blood pressure above the 95th percentile.

Let us look at one more example. As part of a clinical trial evaluating the benefits of tonsillectomy in preventing recurrent throat infections, an informative natural history study was performed.[11] The authors set stringent criteria for entry into their controlled trial of operative procedures. Included was documentation of at least 7 episodes of throat infection in the year prior to entry into the study, 5 episodes in each of the preceding 2 years, or 3 episodes in each of the 3 years prior to study. Of some 300 children evaluated, 95 had histories of recurrent throat infections that met the standards, but they lacked sufficient documentation for inclusion. Generally, this meant that parents reported the problem, but it was not confirmed by a physician or health worker. Sixty-five of these children were followed for a year to see what their natural history of subsequent throat infections would be. Results showed that only 11 of the 65 had a sufficient number of throat infections in the follow-up year to qualify for tonsillectomy. Overall, the group had many fewer throat infections during the observation year than had previously been reported. This is a rather provocative finding since, for this group of children at least, an operation performed at the time of enrollment might well have been credited for the subsequent decline in throat infections. As it is, the authors attribute the findings to natural reduction in illness as children get older and a

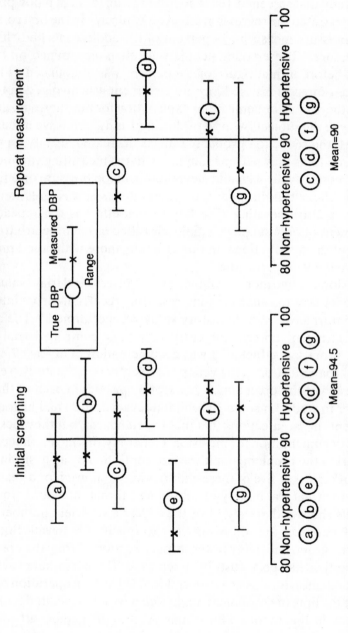

FIGURE 7-6 Regression to the mean in a blood pressure (BP) screening program. Measured pressures (x) in initial screening misclassify subjects c and g as hypertensive. Mean for "hypertensives" (c,d,f,g) is 94.5 mmHg. On repeat measurement, c and g are closer to their true BPs (O). Mean for c,d,f, and g falls to 90 mmHg; b is misclassified as nonhypertensive but never has repeat measurement.

certain unreliability in parents' estimates of past morbidity. Problems with the changing natural history and observer bias are possible. However, there is also a regression effect. In this instance, children have been selected for study only if they have experienced a very high number of throat infections. They are out on the tail of the sore-throat-frequency distribution. Children who have been selected on the basis of seven episodes of throat infection in a single year are likely, on statistical grounds alone, to have fewer episodes in a subsequent year.

The regression effect can occur anytime clinical or laboratory measurements are made on groups of people and individuals are selected for further study on the basis of cut points made on ends of a distribution. Readers need to be aware of this phenomenon since, as is illustrated by the hypertension and sore-throat examples, statistical regression can easily be interpreted as therapeutic benefit. An understanding of the problem suggests its remedy. Before a classification is made, multiple measurements should be obtained to gain a more reliable estimate of the true value in that particular case. Knowledgeable investigators studying hypertension, for example, will take three or four pretreatment blood pressures to establish an estimate of the patient's true blood pressure before any classification or intervention is undertaken. When this precaution is not observed, let the reader beware!

SUMMARY

The problems of making reliable and valid measurements are compounded when measurements are misrepresented or misinterpreted in frequency distributions. The following questions are of particular relevance for readers to ask:

1. How are distributions of data summarized? Are distributions that are likely to be skewed assumed to be normal? When arithmetic means are employed to describe central tendency, do they summarize the data fairly? Are estimates of variability given when data are presented?

2. Are statistical distributions used to define clinical disease? When normal distributions become arbiters of health and

disease, watch out! What is the health status of people on whom reference distributions are created? Are any clinical features used to support arbitrary cutoffs as indicators of disease?

3. Is regression to the mean occurring? If extremes of frequency distributions are used to classify subjects, has care been taken to avoid misclassification? Will subsequent measurements tend to regress and spuriously suggest a treatment effect?

REFERENCES

1. Elveback LR, Guillier CL, Keating FR Jr: Health, normality, and the ghost of Gauss. *JAMA* 211:69, 1970.
2. Gillenwater JY, Harrison RB, Kunin CM: Natural history of bacteriuria in schoolgirls: A long-term case-control study. *N Engl J Med* 301:396, 1979.
3. Barton LL, Feigin RD: Childhood cervical lymphadenitis: A reappraisal. *J Pediatr* 84:846, 1974.
4. Murphy EA, Abbey H: The normal range—A common misuse. *J Chron Dis* 20:79, 1967.
5. Murphy EA: The normal, and the perils of the sylleptic argument. *Perspect Biol Med* 15:566, 1972.
6. Murphy EA: The normal. *Am J Epidemiol* 98:403, 1973.
7. Feinstein AR: *Clinical Biostatistics.* St Louis, Mosby, 1977.
8. Sackett DL: The usefulness of laboratory tests in health-screening programs. *Clin Chem* 19:366, 1973.
9. Fixler DE, Laird WP, Fitzgerald V, et al: Hypertension screening in schools: Results of the Dallas study. *Pediatrics* 63:32, 1979.
10. Sells CJ: Microcephaly in a normal school population. *Pediatrics* 59:262, 1977.
11. Paradise JL, Bluestone CD, Bachman RZ, et al. History of recurrent sore throat as an indication for tonsillectomy: Predictive limitations of histories that are undocumented. *N Engl J Med* 298:409, 1978.

CHAPTER EIGHT

INTERPRETATION: STATISTICAL SIGNIFICANCE

There are three kinds of lies: lies, damn lies, and statistics.

DISRAELI

$\mathcal{M}$r. Disraeli's discomfort with statistics is shared by many clinicians. Somehow the brief exposure to the biostatistics courses offered in college or medical school seems woefully inadequate. A working understanding of p values, chi squares, and the null hypothesis is difficult to come by and easily lost. The current sophistication of statistical presentations in journal articles makes it tempting to abdicate responsibility for interpretations of statistical significance to the statisticians and editors, but that is probably not a wise plan.

For the most part, biostatistics and clinical research work well together. Testing for statistical significance keeps overly optimistic clinical anecdotes in a proper perspective, but there are instances where the fit is not good and the clinical message of the study is drowned in a statistical flood. In this chapter, we will explore the principles underlying the use of tests of statistical significance, clarify some statistical terminology, and look at some common, subtle (and usually unintentional) statistical traps that await the unwary reader.

INFERENCE

To understand statistical significance, we need to know about making inferences. An inference is a generalization made about a large group or population from the study of a sample of that population. To illustrate, suppose you have just completed Saturday morning house calls and stopped by Pritchard's country store to take in a Dr. Pepper and some rural wisdom. Behind the flour sack on which you perch are two apple barrels: one holds red Jonathans, the other, Golden Delicious (to which you are partial). Unfortunately, there has been some mixing of the two varieties, so the red-apple barrel has some goldens in it and vice versa. Proprietor Pritchard, always keen for a wager, says he will give you your favorite if you correctly identify the red-apple and golden-apple barrels by examining only five apples. You reach back, extract the apples from one of the barrels and, finding that one is red and four are yellow, announce that you have found the golden-apple barrel.

You've just made an inferential statement, that is, a judgment about a characteristic of a population (the composition of a whole barrel of apples) from evaluating a sample of the population (5 apples). Simple enough. However, there is a chance that you are wrong. The proportions of your sample may not reflect the composition of the entire barrel. You may have chanced to pick the only four yellow apples in the entire red-apple barrel, made an incorrect inference, and lost the bet. To reduce the likelihood of making an error, your best strategy would be to enlarge the size of your sample. Instead of 5 apples, you could examine 20; or you could increase your sample to 50 or 100 apples. As you come closer to counting the entire barrel of apples, your chance of making a mistaken inference decreases. If, finally, you study all the apples, you are no longer making an inference, and you can be certain of the composition of the barrel.

Most medical studies, whether testing the efficacy of steroids in treating poison ivy dermatitis or looking for an association between exposure to asbestos and occurrence of lung tumors, evaluate samples of larger populations. We examine 50 patients, 200 workers in a single industrial plant, or even an entire community, hoping to generalize about all patients, all chemical plants, or society at large; and as with picking apples at the country store, there is a chance that we will be misled by our sample.

SAMPLING VARIABILITY

Let us suppose we are interested in testing the claim that the antibiotic amoxicillin causes less diarrhea than ampicillin, its cousin. We begin by giving amoxicillin to 50 patients in our practice. We ask the patients to report any episodes of diarrhea that occur while they are taking the medication. It turns out that 6 patients (12 percent) report diarrhea. So far, so good. We would like to be able to predict the behavior of all patients who receive amoxicillin. To verify our earlier results, we select another sample of 50 patients and repeat the experiment. This time only 8 percent of patients experience the side effect. Repeating the experiment yet a third time reveals an incidence of diarrhea of 10 percent.

In attempting to delineate the true incidence of diarrhea for all patients who receive the drug, making inferences from samples of 50, we have uncovered the problem of sampling variability. Each estimate we gather is at slight variance from its predecessor. If we continue repeating our samples of 50 patients, we will find that our collection of results begins to form a pattern. Values begin to cluster around certain recurrent percentages. The results group around 10 percent, which is not only the most common result (the *mode*) but is located in the center of the distribution (the *median*). We find some estimates both higher and lower than 10 percent, but these become less frequent as they become more extreme.

If we had nothing better to do than continue taking our samples of 50 patients over and over, we would form a sampling distribution for the incidence of diarrhea among people given amoxicillin. Figure 8-1 illustrates what this distribution might look like. The conclusion we draw from examining the distribution is that the true incidence of this side effect is about 10 percent, with the understanding that any estimate we make from a single sample of 50 patients may be slightly off the mark. We can examine the plot of diarrhea frequencies and estimate how often we would find a rate as high as 16 percent or as low as 4 percent. Assuming that our experiments are performed reliably, we can predict that this will occur relatively infrequently—about 1 in 20 times.

We still have not answered the question of whether amoxicillin has a lower frequency of diarrhea associated with its use than does ampicillin. Let us find another group of 50 patients, subject them to ampicillin treatment, and ask for reports of diarrhea. The patients provide us with the information that 16 percent of them encountered the side

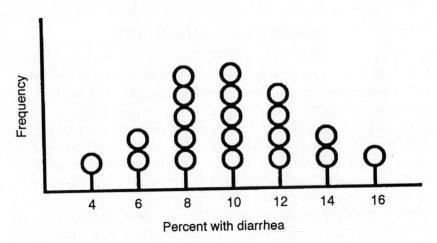

FIGURE 8-1 Percent of patients receiving amoxicillin who develop diarrhea. Based on 20 samples of 50 patients each.

effect. That is an apparent increase over the 10 percent figure we calculated for amoxicillin, but we did note that, occasionally, sampling variability would produce an estimate as high as 16 percent for the frequency of amoxicillin-induced diarrhea. Does the rate we have found for our single sample of ampicillin patients represent a true difference from amoxicillin or have we drawn the 1-in-20 sample from the high end of the same distribution?

THE NULL HYPOTHESIS AND STATISTICAL SIGNIFICANCE

To help answer the question, we need to invoke a major nemesis—the *null hypothesis*. Lack of understanding of just how the null hypothesis operates is the cause of countless headaches. It is different from a research hypothesis. The proposition that amoxicillin causes less diarrhea than ampicillin is a research hypothesis. We expect that by comparing the two drugs, we will find a difference in the incidence of this side effect. The null hypothesis states that there is no difference to be found between the items being compared—in this instance, the two drugs. The null hypothesis is strictly a statistical convention, used for helping us decide how likely it is that our results have been produced by quirks of sampling.

Testing for statistical significance using the null hypothesis has been likened to the judicial process of assuming innocence until guilt is proven. We make the assumption (contrary to our research hypothesis) that the true incidence of diarrhea for the two preparations is no different: Ampicillin is innocent of causing more diarrhea. Taking on the role of prosecuting attorney, we then try to demonstrate beyond reasonable doubt that in fact there is a difference. *Rejecting* the null hypothesis supports the research hypothesis.

We know that repeating the amoxicillin experiment on 50 people would yield a result of 16 percent incidence of diarrhea only 1 in 20 times. That is a reasonably unlikely occurrence. So when we learn that ampicillin causes diarrhea in 16 percent of patients in our single sample, we have useful evidence to argue. We can say that if ampicillin really behaved like amoxicillin, it would be unlikely (a 5 percent chance) that we would find a 16 percent rate of diarrhea in a single sample. This 5 percent probability is referred to as the *p* value. It is the likelihood of obtaining our result if the null hypothesis were true. We feel that a 1-in-20 chance is too small to continue to support the null hypothesis, so we reject it and proclaim that our findings are "statistically significant": the drugs cause diarrhea at different rates.

Most often, results of clinical studies are said to be statistically significant, that is, unlikely to be due to chance, if the *p* value is less than 5 percent (.05) or 1 percent (.01). But there is nothing magical about these levels of probability. The .05 tradition began in the 1920s with an influential statistician named Fisher. It has been habit ever since. Frequently we read articles in which a wide variety of *p* values is used, ranging from .05 to values that are many times smaller. Small *p* values like .001 or .0001 are important to the extent that they tell us that differences we observe are unlikely to be mistakes in inference due to sampling, but we need to be wary of a subtle illusion that is created by these impressive numbers.

SOME PROBLEMS OF STATISTICAL SIGNIFICANCE

The size of the p value does not indicate the importance of the result   It is tempting to believe that very small *p* values indicate great discoveries. Terms such as "highly significant results" and "very highly significant results" are liberally sprinkled through journals. Consider an article that demonstrated a correlation between alcohol consumption and elevated blood pressure.[1] In this study, the amount of daily intake of alcoholic beverages was compared with blood pressure readings for patients in a prepaid group practice. A difference in average blood pressure was found between individuals who drank small amounts of alcohol and those with high intake. Those who drank more had higher blood pressure. This finding was reported as statistically significant, with a p value of 10^{-24}. Extraordinary! Enough "highlys" in that significant result to cover an entire page. But what does this value really mean? Simply that the difference found is not likely to have occurred because of sampling alone. It does not mean that the findings are of major medical importance, nor does it mean that alcohol consumption is a major cause of hypertension. It means only that chance is an unlikely explanation for the results. This extremely small p value is due to the size of the sample, 80,000 people in all. Very large samples become close approximations of the populations they are estimating, so any differences that are found are likely to be real (like examining all the apples in the barrel). There is little reason to report such an absurd p value. The results are scarcely more credible than had they been achieved with a value of 1 in 10,000. Yet it is difficult for a reader not to be awed by such a statistical tour de force, even though it adds nothing of substance to the study.

Results may be statistically significant but clinically unimportant Just as it is easy to be impressed by small p values, so can we be seduced into equating statistical significance with clinical importance. Consider a frequently referenced article on the therapy of otitis media.[2] In this clinical trial, the authors compare the efficacy of several drugs commonly used in treating ear infections. Among the drugs tested was an antihistamine. In comparing the responses of patients prescribed the antihistamine with those not treated, a statistically significant reduction in treatment failures was found when the antihistamine was used. The results of the study are summarized in Table 8-1. It is easy to conclude that antihistamines should be used in the treatment of otitis media. Let us examine these data more closely.

The number of children treated with the antihistamine was 250; the number left untreated was about the same. For the treated group,

· TABLE 8-1 ·		
Failure rates for patients with otitis media treated with and without antihistamines		
	With antihistamines	**Without antihistamines**
Patients treated	250	264
Treatment failures	4 (1.6%)	13 (4.9%)

SOURCE: Modified from Stickler et al.[2]

there was a failure rate of approximately 2 percent, compared with a 5 percent rate for those left untreated. This twofold difference in failure rates is indeed statistically significant; it would have occurred only 5 in 100 times by chance. The question remains, however, is the treatment clinically important? Among the 514 children who had ear infections, only 9 treatment failures were prevented by the use of the medication. Is this benefit dramatic enough to warrant large-scale deployment of antihistamines as a major weapon against otitis? Probably not.

To learn more about the outcome of primary-care residency training programs, a group of investigators tracked career choice, board certification, and practice location for groups of internal medicine and pediatrics residency graduates.[3] Comparisons were made between doctors trained in "traditional" and "primary-care" programs. One finding that was featured in the article's abstract was that "board certification rates in internal medicine were statistically higher for graduates of primary care training programs (80%) than for graduates of traditional programs (76%, $p=.002$) but were not statistically significant for both groups of pediatric graduates."[3] Here, another small p value seems portentous. But how important are these results? Table 8-2 elaborates on the data.

It turns out that the 80 to 76 percent differential in certification rates found among internal medicine graduates is exactly reversed for pediatricians. Eighty percent of traditional program grads are certified, compared with 76 percent of those from the primary-care residency. Why should the same percentage-point difference prompt a significant p value for internists while leaving pediatricians out? Three times as many internists were included in this study as pediatricians and sheer force of numbers enabled the authors to reject the null

• TABLE 8-2 •		
Percentage of graduates of internal medicine and pediatrics training programs who are board-certified		
	Percent certified, number of graduates	
	Internal medicine[a]	**Pediatrics**[b]
Traditional training	76 (12,594)	80 (3,411)
Primary-care training	80 (1,156)	76 (772)

[a]Difference between traditional and primary-care training statistically significant ($p=.002$).
[b]Difference between traditional and primary-care training not statistically significant ($p =.089$).
SOURCE: Adapted from Noble et al.[3]

hypothesis in one instance but not in the other. In fact, the small difference in certification rates is of no real importance. In discussing results, the authors even point to the group *similarities* as evidence of comparable preparation from the training tracks. Somewhere along the way, the glint of the significant *p* value proved too alluring and a statistically significant but practically unimportant result became a prominent part of the abstract.

Differences that are not statistically significant are not necessarily unimportant We have already agreed that most medical researchers look for differences and that rejecting the null hypothesis "proves" the difference. However, failure to reject the null hypothesis does not guarantee that differences observed are not real or that the groups being compared are the same. Another study of otitis media illustrates the point.

Roddey et al. designed a clinical trial to test whether myringotomies aided the resolution of ear infections.[4] To a standard antibiotic regimen they randomly added the minor operative procedure for one-half the patients. Among children having myringotomies, a treatment failure rate of 24 percent was found, compared with 35 percent for those in whom the procedure was not performed (see Table 8-3). The difference just missed statistical significance at the chosen *p* value of .05; for the number of children observed, quirks of sampling could produce the same difference between 5 percent and 10 percent of the time. That was not enough evidence for Roddey to win his case and

• TABLE 8-3 • Failure rates for patients with otitis media treated with and without myringotomy		
	With myringotomy	Without myringotomy
Patients treated	113	127
Treatment failures	27 (24%)	44 (35%)

SOURCE: Modified from Roddey et al.[4]

reject the null hypothesis. The findings might be due to chance. These conclusions have been summarized in subsequent articles as demonstrating that "myringotomy made no difference in the resolution of otitis media." This is not really true. Roddey found a difference. In fact, myringotomy prevented more treatment failures (11 per 100 patients) than did the use of antihistamines (3 per 100 patients). Sample size is again the key. Had Roddey studied the same number of patients as were in the antihistamine trial and found the same 11 percentage points difference in failure rate, his results would have been statistically significant. As it is, we can only say that the fewer treatment failures found after myringotomy might have been an artifact of sampling.

When Savard-Fenton et al.[5] compared the efficacy of single-dose with multidose amoxicillin treatment for uncomplicated urinary tract infection (UTI), they employed the null hypothesis to help interpret results. However, in this study, significance testing was not intended to show that the treatments differ in efficacy but that they are equivalent. The researchers randomly allocated 388 women with symptoms of UTI to receive either one 3-g dose of amoxicillin or 250 mg of the drug three times daily for 2 weeks. Among the 162 patients with bacteriologically confirmed infections who returned at 1 week for follow-up cultures, 71 had received the single-dose and 91 the 2-week treatment. Cure rates were 60.6 and 73.6 percent, respectively. How should this difference of 13 percentage points in cure rates be interpreted? Are the rates estimates from two different populations of responses? Or could the difference be due to sampling variability, and the two estimates really represent the same "true" cure rate?

The authors performed a test of significance and found a p value of .07. This p value was not small enough for them to reject the null hypothesis and say that the cure rates differed, so they concluded that "a single three gram dose of amoxicillin, with follow-up urine culture, provides safe and effective management for acute, uncomplicated urinary tract infections in non-pregnant women."[5] Still, we are uneasy that the 13 percent difference in cure rates could be clinically important. If the study sample had included 200 patients equally divided between the two groups instead of 162, and the same cure rates obtained, the p value would be .05 and the conclusion might have been different.

BETA ERRORS AND STATISTICAL POWER

Two kinds of mistakes can be made in the search for statistical significance. The first occurs when we reject the null hypothesis and it is true. We claim that two treatments are dissimilar and, in fact, they are no different. This is an alpha, or type I, error and occurs when we claim different rates of diarrhea for ampicillin and amoxicillin when, in fact, the drugs behave no differently. The second potential hypothesis-testing error is suggested in the example of myringotomy and otitis media. Failing to reject the null hypothesis when it is not true is a beta, or type II, mistake. A true treatment effect or difference is being overlooked. Table 8-4 schematizes the correct and incorrect decisions that can be

		Null hypothesis (treatment A = treatment B)	
		True (no difference)	**False** (difference)
Decision (based on statistical test)	**Accept** (No difference)	Correct	Type II, beta error
	Reject (Difference)	Type I, alpha error	Correct

• TABLE 8-4 •
Errors encountered in testing the null hypothesis to evaluate efficacy of treatments A and B

reached when we are testing the null hypothesis. Rejecting the notion that two treatments are identical when they are different and finding no difference when none exists are correct decisions. Of the incorrect conclusions, the alpha error is most familiar to clinicians. We worry about claiming that a new treatment is effective when chance could have produced the difference we observe. We are accustomed to seeing *p* values, and conceptualization of this first type of error is reasonably straightforward.

Coming to an understanding of beta errors is a bit trickier. We wish to avoid making the mistake of missing a therapeutic effect; that is, of accepting the idea that two treatments are the same simply because we cannot reject the null hypothesis and state that they are different. But, once we start speaking of rejecting and accepting differences, the question becomes, "Differences of what size?" Roddey found an 11 percent difference in cure rate between his myringotomy group and controls.[4] He might have observed a difference of 8, 2, or 16 percent. The range of possibilities is infinite. When we speak of the likelihood of missing a treatment effect in our hypothesis testing, the size of the difference we are looking for is crucial. For each possible difference that might exist, there is a different probability of making a beta error. The whole business of beta error is an interplay between the magnitude of difference, the number of subjects involved, and the alpha level at which experimenters decide they will reject the null hypothesis.

Researchers can lessen their chances of making beta errors by altering these three basic ingredients. We speak of the process of reducing beta error as improving experimental power. Statistical power is the complement of beta error (power $= 1 -$ beta error); the lower the beta error, the greater the power. The power of an experiment is the likelihood that the experiment will detect a treatment effect of a particular size (a difference) for a particular number of experimental subjects. The higher the power, the better our chances of finding the treatment benefit, if it is there. The most obvious way of increasing power is to increase the number of subjects studied. If Roddey had studied twice the number of subjects and found the same 11 percent difference, it would have been statistically significant (it would have occurred by chance less than 5 percent of the time). Power is also influenced by the size of the difference. For a given number of subjects, an experiment will have a higher probability of detecting a large treatment effect than a small difference. A 50 percent difference in cure rates for the original numbers of myringotomy and control subjects would have a high probability of leading to rejection of the null hypothesis. Power may also be improved if we are willing to raise the alpha level. Roddey's findings would have been statistically significant at an alpha level of 10 percent. But to increase the likelihood of finding a statistically significant difference by changing alpha, we must also increase the possibility of falsely claiming an experiment effect. Comfort with these concepts requires some pondering, but they are worth trying to master. Several discussions of the topic are available.[6,7]

Ideally, power calculations should be made before an experiment is performed. Investigators should decide on the number of subjects they require on the basis of estimates of the size of the difference they wish to detect and the certainty with which they desire to pinpoint that difference. In general, a power of 80 to 90 percent is considered respectable. However, things do not always work out that way.

Freiman and colleagues analyzed 71 studies from major medical journals that reported negative results; that is, no difference was found between treatments studied.[7] The investigators found that a high percentage of these studies could have missed an important difference in therapies because an inadequate number of subjects was evaluated. Many of the studies actually showed trends suggesting that a treatment worked, but the authors concluded that the therapy was no different from control simply because they could not reject the null hypothesis. Results reported in experimental and observational studies may be negative not because there are no differences but because the power of the study was too low to detect meaningful differences. Researchers should comment about power when they present negative results. They should provide some estimate of the probability that, for the number of subjects studied and the alpha level considered reasonable for rejecting the null hypothesis, a meaningful difference between groups would have been detected. Presenting confidence intervals is also of help.

CONFIDENCE INTERVALS

Many now feel that the *confidence interval* (CI) gives readers more useful information than the *p* value alone. The value of *p* provides a standardized estimate of the likelihood that we would encounter differences as large as or larger than those we have discovered if there were actually no difference or effect (the null hypothesis were true). But we do not learn anything about the size of the result itself. When CI reporting is used, a point estimate of the result is given together with a range of values that are also consistent with the data at hand. When this range is large, many possible results must be considered— some much greater than the estimate provided by the study, some much smaller. Sometimes the CI includes *zero* difference between two therapies or *no* risk associated with an exposure, and we must concede that corticosteroids may not benefit meningitis patients or caffeine intake lead to heart attack.

When Savard-Fenton et al.[5] tested the difference in cure rates between single-dose and 2-week therapy for UTI (60.6 and 73.6 percent, respectively), they obtained a *p* value of .07. On this basis they could not reject the null hypothesis at the 5 percent level. So they suggested that their cure rates were statistically equivalent. There was, however, a difference of 13 percentage points between the two treatments. When a 95 percent CI for this 13 percent cure rate difference is calculated, the range extends from −1.5 to 27.5 percent. In other words, the 13-percentage-point advantage of 2-week therapy is the best point estimate of difference we can obtain from this single study. But the investigators' data are consistent with differences anywhere in the CI from 1.5 percent in favor of single-dose to 27.5 percent in favor of 2-week therapy. The CI includes zero difference, which is the reason the investigators were unable to reject the null hypothesis. In general, when a 95 percent CI contains a zero difference, it is equivalent to saying that one is unable to reject the null hypothesis at the 5 percent level. Wide CIs indicate greater uncertainty about the true value of a result; a smaller CI narrows the reasonable choices. Several journals have published useful discussions about CIs,[8–11] including their use to assess clinical and statistical significance at the same time.[12]

TESTING FOR STATISTICAL SIGNIFICANCE MAY BE IRRELEVANT

Bearing in mind that significance testing simply tells us the likelihood of finding results because of sampling variability, we can find examples of studies where chance is not really at issue. In a study of the effect of weight reduction on the blood pressure of overweight, hypertensive patients,[13] information is presented comparing weight loss among dieting patients and a nondieting control group. Of 81 patients who were dieting, every patient lost weight; the lowest loss reported was 3 kg and the average about 9 kg. The control group underwent very little change in weight, losing less than a kilogram on average. In assessing these findings the authors note, "this reduction was highly significant...$p < .001$." Of course, there is nothing really wrong with this statistical claim. However, the finding is so obvious that it scarcely merits statistical enforcement. We do not need a p value to tell us that patients who adhere to a diet and uniformly lose weight differ from nondieting controls.

Studies sometimes employ statistics that give an appearance of profundity while illustrating the obvious. In an article on the prevention of injuries to children in automobiles,[14] a series of 200 roadside observations was made of safety practices and their relationship to other "characteristics of the journey." A positive relationship was found between children riding in the rear seat (a good safety practice) and the number of adults riding in the automobile. This finding is reported as statistically significant at the $p < .001$ level. Impressive! But at second glance, it is hardly an insight likely to revolutionize highway safety. The percentage of children in the back seat rises as the number of adults in the automobile increases. Children have to sit somewhere, and since adults usually lay claim to the front seat, the kids get displaced to the back. Attaching a fancy p value to trivial observations does little to enhance their importance.

Alternate explanations of the observed difference

Having observed differences that are statistically significant, we are tempted to conclude that our treatments or theories are responsible for observed effects. Unfortunately, this may not be true. Remember, when we reject the null hypothesis, we only assess the role chance may have played in creating differences.

Capricious methodology may still be at play. The many systematic biases—like the subject-allocation bias seen in the birthing-room experiment[15] or the selective recall of the accident-prone aviators—could account for results. The increased survival of heart-attack patients who participated in the exercise program[16] and high incidence of abuse and neglect reported among children identified in the nursery as at risk[17] were statistically significant findings, but biases in both studies may make statistical proclamations superfluous. The British statistician Sir Austin Bradford Hill has remarked that too often "the glitter of the t-table diverts attention from the inadequacies of the fare."[18]

SUMMARY

Statistical tests need to be kept in proper perspective. Tests of significance tell us about the role that sampling variability may have played in results. They make no other claim on the validity of the study. All our concerns about the effects of sampling procedures, proper measurement, and the many opportunities for bias still pertain. Readers who can keep their heads when those about them are lost in a swirl of p values have an advantage. They can concentrate on issues of relevance.

Ask the following:

1. Are the differences observed between the groups under study likely to be due to chance?

2. If differences are not due to chance, do they occur because of biases or are they related to the treatment or another study factor?

3. If differences are statistically significant (not due to chance), are they clinically important?

4. If differences are not statistically significant, is it possible that a true difference has been overlooked (a type II error made)?

REFERENCES

1. Klatsky AL, Friedman GD, Siegelaub AB, Gerard MJ: Alcohol consumption and blood pressure. *N Engl J Med* 296:1194, 1977.

2. Stickler GB, Rubenstein MM, McBean JB et al: Treatment of acute otitis media in children: IV. A fourth clinical trial. *Am J Dis Child* 114:123, 1967.
3. Noble J, Friedman RH, Starfield B, et al: Career differences between primary care and traditional trainees in internal medicine and pediatrics. *Ann Intern Med* 116:482, 1992.
4. Roddey OF Jr, Earle R Jr, Haggerty R: Myringotomy in acute otitis media: A controlled study. *JAMA* 197:849, 1966.
5. Savard-Fenton M, Fenton BW, Reller LB et al: Single-dose amoxicillin therapy with follow-up urine culture: Effective initial management for acute uncomplicated urinary tract infections. *Am J Med* 73:808, 1982.
6. Berwick DM: Experimental power: The other side of the coin. *Pediatrics* 65:1043, 1980.
7. Freiman JA, Chalmers TC, Smith H, Kuebler RR: The importance of beta, the type II error and sample size in the design and interpretation of the randomized control trial: Survey of 71 "negative" trials. *N Engl J Med* 299:690, 694, 1978.
8. Bulpitt CJ: Confidence intervals. *Lancet* 1:494, 1987.
9. Confidence intervals extract clinically useful information from data, editorial. *Ann Intern Med* 108:296, 1988.
10. Gardner MJ, Altman DG: Confidence intervals rather than P values: Estimation rather than hypothesis testing. *Br Med J* 292:746, 1986.
11. Rothman KJ: A show of confidence. *N Engl J Med* 299:1362, 1978.
12. Braitman LE: Confidence intervals assess both clinical significance and statistical significance. *Ann Intern Med* 114:515, 1991.
13. Reisin E, Abel R, Modan M, et al: Effect of weight loss without salt restriction on the reduction of blood pressure in overweight hypertensive patients. *N Engl J Med* 298:1, 1978.
14. Pless IB, Roghmann K, Algranati P: The prevention of injuries to children in automobiles. *Pediatrics* 49:420, 1972.
15. Goodlin RC: Low-risk obstetric care for low-risk mothers. *Lancet* 1:1017, 1980.
16. Rechnitzer PA, Pickard HA, Paivio AU, et al: Long-term follow-up study of survival and recurrence rates following myocardial infarction in exercising and control subjects. *Circulation* 45:853, 1972.
17. Hunter RS, Kilstrom N, Kraybill EN, Loda F: Antecedents of child abuse and neglect in premature infants: A prospective study in a newborn intensive care unit. *Pediatrics* 61:629, 1978.
18. Hill AB: The environment and disease: Association or causation? *Proc Roy Soc Med* 58:295, 1965.

CHAPTER NINE

INTERPRETATION: SOME STATISTICAL TESTS

A student set forth on a quest,
To learn which of the world's beers was best,
But his wallet was dried out
At the first pub he tried out,
With two samples he flunked the means test.

The type of statistical maneuver an author chooses depends upon properties of the data that need to be analyzed, how the data are distributed, and what questions they are to answer. Statisticians speak of four types of data: nominal, ordinal, interval, and ratio. *Nominal* data are, as the appellation implies, named categories. ABO blood groups, male or female sex, treatment cures or failures are examples. These have no mathematical relationship to one another; they are neither ranked nor ordered. Sometimes numbers or letters are used to identify categories, such as license plate numbers, numbers on baseball uniforms, or designations such as diabetes type I or type II. Though these numbers may be convenient as identifying symbols, it must be remembered that they are only symbols with no mathematical properties. They cannot legitimately be added or subtracted from one another. From an analytical point of view, each is a separate entity having an equivalent weight or value.

Ordinal data can be sequenced or ranked—smallest to largest, lightest to heaviest, easiest to most difficult, "always agree" to "never agree." Examples include socioeconomic classes, military grades, academic ranks, medical conditions (such as stable to critical), or health-status indicators (such as excellent, good, fair, and poor). These represent ranks, but the distances or intervals between the categories are not necessarily uniform. It is clear to most everyone that excellent health is preferred to good health and that good health is better than "fair" or "poor" health. But how much better is excellent than good? Is the difference between good health and fair health the same as the difference between fair health and poor health? One cannot say. The order is understood, but the intervals between classes are not defined and cannot be assumed to be equivalent.

That claim can only be made for *interval* and *ratio* data. These share the properties of having rank or order, but they also have known, equal distances between values. Ratio data have a true zero point as well as equal intervals, but this distinction is not a major sticking point for most of the statistical testing encountered in our reading. We will speak of interval and ratio data together as *continuous* data. Temperature, height, weight, and blood sugar concentration share the properties of equal intervals. The distance between 33° and 34°C is the same as that from 39° to 40°C. The loss of 2 g of hemoglobin is the same, whether the level drops from 16 to 14 g or from 10 to 8 g (even though the clinical implications may not be the same).

Continuous data lend themselves readily to arithmetic operations such as addition and subtraction, and if there is a true zero in the interval scale (kilograms, inches, hematocrit), multiplication and division are possible. Data of this sort can be averaged to give the mean height for eighth-grade girls from Spokane or the mean and standard deviation blood lead level for workers in a battery warehouse.

Nominal and ordinal data must be handled more gingerly. Because they are categorical and lack mathematical equivalence, they cannot legitimately be added or subtracted. Different types of statistical tests are appropriate.

To make the world of statistical tests a bit less foreign, let us look at some examples of several of the most commonly used statistical approaches to analyzing medical data. The objective here is not to become proficient in performing these tests but to gain an intuitive feel for how the data are being handled. For those who need a more detailed understanding, resources are available.[1,2]

Let us suppose that we are conducting an experiment in our practice to find a remedy for the many patients who come in complaining of fatigue. Over the years, we have noted that several remedies appear useful, but we have never subjected them to the close scrutiny that our increasingly critical sensibilities tell us is required. Two treatments come to mind: Lydia Pinkham's Compound and Bull Durham's Liver Extract. Accordingly, we approach the next 80 patients who visit with the chief complaint of "feeling tired" and ask them to participate in our study. All willingly agree to be randomly allocated to one of the two treatments. They consent to swallow a teaspoonful of either Lydia Pinkham's Compound or Bull Durham's Liver Extract three times a day for the next 2 weeks. Naturally, we have made certain that the two tonics look and taste the same and that the bottles are labeled with a study number to which only a pharmacist friend has the identifying key. After patients have completed the full course of treatment, we quiz them about any change in level of energy, classifying each into one of three categories: much peppier, somewhat peppier, or not improved.

Of the 80 patients we enroll, 42 are randomized to the Lydia Pinkham group and 38 are dosed with Bull Durham. Patient outcomes are seen in Table 9-1. Inspection of the table suggests that more patients improved with Lydia Pinkham's than with Bull Durham's, but some patients in each group are much improved and some failed to improve at all. Is Lydia Pinkham's superior to Bull Durham's in relieving fatigue?

· **TABLE 9-1** ·

Condition of patients after receiving Lydia Pinkham's Compound or Bull Durham's Extract—observed values

	No. of patients			
Treatment	Much peppier	Somewhat peppier	Not improved	Total
Lydia Pinkham's	14	19	9	42
Bull Durham's	9	11	18	38
Total:	23	30	27	80

Tests for Categorical Data

The test most commonly used for these categorical kinds of data is called the *chi-square test*. The chi-square statistic takes the distribution of results (much peppier, somewhat peppier, and not improved) for the two samples (Lydia Pinkham's and Bull Durham's) and gives us an estimate of the likelihood that these two samples are representative of the overall population. What is the distribution of all fatigued people who report their state of energy 2 weeks after a course of medication? Are our two treatment distributions different enough from one another that they are not likely to have been drawn from the same parent population? Are the differences we observe real or simply an artifact of sampling variability?

To answer this question, we need some notion of the "true" population values. Our best approximation from the data at hand is the number of patients in each category from the total number of subjects in our study—the combined sample of patients given Lydia Pinkham's and Bull Durham's. These figures are seen in the bottom row of Table 9-1, the "bottom marginal." Among all our patients, 23 reported feeling much peppier, 30 were somewhat peppier, and 27 remained unimproved. The chi-square test uses these marginal values as an estimate of the population, or as *expected* values if no differences existed between the treatment groups. The *observed* number of cases in each cell is compared with the number that would be expected on the basis of the distribution of the bottom marginal. Each expected value is calculated by multiplying the total number of patients in each treatment group by the proportion of each outcome represented in the bottom row of each column (Table 9-2). The difference between each observed and expected value is squared, divided by the particular expected value, and summed to give the value of chi square. This number is matched with a standard table of chi-square values to determine the probability that the collection of observed and expected differences could be explained by chance. The larger the difference between what we observe and what we expect, the larger the value of chi-square and the lower the p value. Table 9-2 shows how a chi-square statistic would be calculated for our experiment. The summed value of 6.09 would occur only 5 in 100 times by chance ($p = .049$), so, according to common practice, we could reject the null hypothesis that the Lydia Pinkham's and Bull Durham's treatments were no different—that is, that the figures are estimates of the same population. We

• TABLE 9-2 •
Condition of patients after receiving Lydia Pinkham's Compound or Bull Durham's Extract—expected values

	Category			
Treatment	**Much peppier**	**Somewhat peppier**	**Not improved**	**Total**
Lydia Pinkham's	$42 \times {}^{23}/_{80} = 12.1$	$42 \times {}^{30}/_{80} = 15.7$	$42 \times {}^{27}/_{80} = 14.2$	42
Bull Durham's	$38 \times {}^{23}/_{80} = \underline{10.9}$	$38 \times {}^{30}/_{80} = \underline{14.3}$	$38 \times {}^{27}/_{80} = \underline{12.8}$	$\underline{38}$
	23	30	27	80

Chi-square = sum of $\dfrac{\text{(observed-expected)}^2}{\text{expected}}$

$$= \frac{(14-12.1)^2}{12.1} + \frac{(19-15.7)^2}{15.7} + \frac{(9-14.2)^2}{14.2} + \frac{(9-10.9)^2}{10.9} + \frac{(11-14.3)^2}{14.3} + \frac{(18-12.8)^2}{12.8}$$

$$= 0.30 + 0.69 + 1.90 + 0.33 + 0.76 + 2.11$$

$$= 6.09, p = .049$$

then conclude that, since we believe our experimental design to have avoided biases that could account for the observed treatment responses, Lydia Pinkham's does a better job than Bull Durham's at pepping up our patients.

Although the chi-square test is the most commonly used of the tests for categorical data, a number of others will be encountered in your reading. *Fisher's exact test* is used for data that can be placed in two-by-two tables—two treatments and two responses. This test is particularly useful when the overall number of subjects is small or if the expected number in any of the cells is small. Some statisticians prefer the exact to the chi-square test in two-by-two situations because, as the name suggests, the exact test estimates exact probabilities of values falling in the cell distributions observed, whereas the chi-square test gives only an approximation.

There are other statistical tests that take advantage of the ordered sequences of categorical data.[3] The outcomes of our Lydia Pinkham–Bull Durham experiment (much peppier, somewhat peppier, and not improved) are ordinal data. However, when we employed the chi-square test, we really treated them as if they were nominal data (equal in value) only; we failed to incorporate the additional information that "much peppier" is better than "somewhat peppier," which is better than "not improved." By failing to take advantage of this useful information, we lost efficiency or power in our statistical testing. We used a lower-octane test when a higher-octane test was available and appropriate. In so doing, we jeopardized our ability to detect a difference between our two treatments when one was indeed present—the type II error we discussed in the previous chapter. Although in this situation chi-square was sufficient to detect a difference in our treatment groups, a shift in the categories of only one or two patients might have lowered the value of chi-square, giving us a slightly higher p value, and we would not have rejected the null hypothesis. Selecting a more powerful test reduces that risk.

TESTS FOR CONTINUOUS DATA

Other statistical maneuvers are available to medical researchers that can legitimately be used only on continuous data under conditions in which the data can be assumed to be normally distributed. The most commonly encountered is the t test, or Student's t, named not because of the delight the procedure evokes among students struggling with statistics but in honor of the British mathematician who developed it. This man's name, as it turns out, was Gossett, and he worked not for any of the prestigious medical research units of Great Britain but for the Guinness Brewery. Guinness employed Gossett to work out statistical sampling techniques that would improve the quality and reproducibility of its beer-making procedures. Gossett published his statistical work under the name of "Student," presumably to keep his trade secrets from the eyes of Guinness competitors.

Student's t test compares the means of two samples of observations to help the researcher (or brewer) decide whether the samples are likely to come from the same or different populations. Anytime continuous data are collected on two groups of subjects, you are likely to find t tests being used. Differences between the blood pressures of patients eating high- and low-sodium diets, or examination scores for students given self-instruction programs instead of lectures, or lengths of hospital stay by patients enrolled in fee-for-service or prepaid insurance programs can all be assessed by using t tests. To construct and interpret a *t* test, one needs to know the size of the samples, the magnitude of differences between the two sample means, and the variability of the data in each sample. When the difference between two means is large, the variability among data is small, and the sample size is reasonably large, the likelihood is increased that the sample means represent two different populations. The summary *t* statistic and its corresponding calculated *p* value can be used as a guide for rejecting the null hypothesis.

To illustrate, let us return to our fatigue experiment. We have a hunch that improvements in fatigue found in our patients who took Lydia Pinkham's Compound have a physiologic basis. We suspect that many of our tired patients are, in fact, suffering from anemia. The magic of Lydia Pinkham's, we hypothesize, is due to its iron content, which raises the hemoglobin level of patients and is responsible for their increased pep. Accordingly, we obtain hemoglobin determinations on patients in both treatment groups at the completion of therapy. The resulting distributions of hemoglobin levels for the Lydia Pinkham's and Bull Durham's patients are displayed in Fig. 9-1. As can be seen from this visual display, the group of Lydia Pinkham's patients appears to have a greater number of higher hemoglobin values. If we calculate posttreatment mean hemoglobin levels for each group by summing the observations and dividing by the total number of subjects, we find that Lydia Pinkham's subjects' average hemoglobin value is 13.6 g, compared with 12.6 g for the Bull Durham's patients. Does this difference of 1 g between the means indicate that the samples represent different populations and that patients who plied themselves with Lydia Pinkham's and reported feeling better have higher levels of hemoglobin? Or is the difference simply due to sampling variability? The *t* test helps answer this.

For the 42 patients who received Lydia Pinkham's Compound, the average posttreatment hemoglobin level was 13.6 g with a standard deviation (measure of variability) of 1.2 g. For the 38 Bull Durham's patients, the mean hemoglobin level was 12.6 g with a standard deviation of 0.8. The *t* value or *t* statistic computed for these data turns out to be 4.0. Checking in the *t* table of a standard statistical text, and using the size of our samples as a guide, we find that the probability (*p* value) of obtaining a *t* value of this magnitude is only .0001. In other words, given the size of our samples and the variability of the data, we would expect to see a difference between estimated means as large as the one we observe only 1 in 10,000 times if the null hypothesis were true and

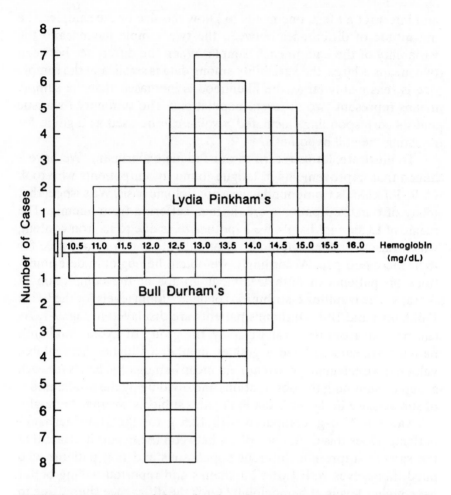

FIGURE 9-1 Hemoglobin levels of patients treated with Lydia Pinkham's Compound and Bull Durham's Extract.

both samples were derived from the same population. Thus, it seems unlikely that sampling variability is responsible for our results, and we decide that in fact our Lydia Pinkham's patients have higher hemoglobin levels than those who received Bull Durham's Extract.

Another way of assessing our result is to construct one of the confidence intervals described in the previous chapter. A 95 percent confidence interval turns out to be 0.5 to 1.4. This means that our estimate for the true difference in hemoglobin levels is consistent with a range between 0.5 and 1.4 g. This interval does not contain 0 g, or no difference, between the groups.

CORRELATION

Correlation is another commonly encountered statistical procedure. *Correlation* evaluates the strength of linear relationships or associations between variables. How closely are patients' weights and blood pressures related to one another? Is the time patients spend in the waiting room linked to their satisfaction? Does the risk of acquiring AIDS increase with the number of blood transfusions a patient receives? With correlation, we observe how the changes in one variable, such as blood pressure or satisfaction, are related to changes in a second measure, such as weight or waiting time. For every incremental increase or decrease in kilograms or minutes spent in the waiting room, is there a predictable increase or decrease in millimeters of mercury of systolic blood pressure or levels of satisfaction on a self-rating questionnaire?

The concept of correlation is depicted graphically in Fig. 9-2. The scatterplot of data in this figure displays a relationship between the variables "weight" on the X axis and "blood pressure" on the Y axis. As x increases in value, so does y. The statistic that summarizes this relationship is called the *correlation coefficient,* symbolized by r. Several tests of correlation are commonly used, depending upon the distribution of data being analyzed. The coefficient characterizes the relationship between the x and y variables. The closer values cluster in a linear relationship, the higher the correlation coefficient and the greater the association between x and y. Correlation coefficients range between -1 and $+1$. If one value decreases while another increases, the coefficient is negative. So r is commonly expressed as .56, $-.10$, and so on. The closer a correlation coefficient is to 1.0 (or to -1.0), the more strongly associated the data. As with other relationships, there are tests to determine whether correlations are "statistically significant." On the basis of the numbers of observations and the variability of the data, how likely is it that the observed association is due to chance? Correlation coefficients are usually reported together with the familiar p value. In the case of the data shown in Fig. 9-2, the Pearson correlation coefficient is .69, indicating a strong, positive relationship between weight and systolic blood pressure. The value of p is less than .001, suggesting that the association is unlikely to be due to quirks of sampling.

As another example, let us examine an observation that several medical students have made that there are differences in the way

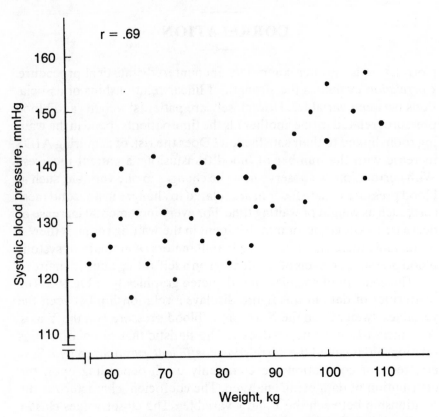

FIGURE 9-2 Systolic blood pressure and weight of 36 patients.

residents and faculty evaluate students on the internal medicine service. The students feel that faculty ratings are heavily influenced by the demonstration of knowledge, while residents consider other aspects of work performance as well. The students are willing to wager that if we compare clinical grades given by faculty and residents with student results on standardized knowledge-based examinations, we will see a strong relationship between performance on the knowledge-based exams and faculty ratings.

Intrigued with this hypothesis, we collect evaluation data on the last 36 students who completed the internal medicine rotation. A partial list of these data is shown in Table 9-3. It is difficult to determine much from data organized in the manner shown in the table, so we construct two scatterplots to help us visualize the relationships. The upper scatterplot in Fig. 9-3 depicts the association between faculty

• TABLE 9-3 •
Clinical ratings of faculty and residents compared with examination scores for 36 students (partial list)

Student	Clinical rating		Examination score
	Faculty	**Resident**	
A	86	90	520
B	85	86	530
C	87	88	445
D	89	85	580
E	94	96	680
F	84	82	430
–	–	–	–
–	–	–	–

grades (on the Y axis) and examination scores (on the X axis); the lower scatterplot shows the data for resident grades and examination scores. Both plots suggest a positive relationship—that higher examination scores are associated with higher clinical grades. However, the points are more tightly clustered and thus the relationship appears to be stronger for faculty grades and exam scores.

This relationship can also be summarized statistically by calculating a correlation coefficient for each set of data. The Pearson coefficient r is .66 for the data depicting faculty grades and examination scores and .21 for the data showing resident grades and examination scores. These coefficients support the associations suggested in the scatterplots. Faculty grading appears more closely related to cognitive examination results than does resident grading. The data support (though certainly do not prove) the students' hypothesis.

REGRESSION

Correlation belongs to a larger class of statistical techniques known as regression. *Regression analysis* works on the principle we have just examined. A line is fitted to a group of data to describe relationships between variables. However, regression analysis can be put to more am-

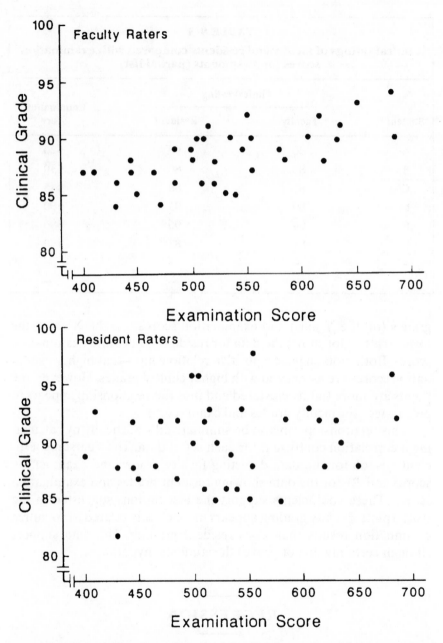

FIGURE 9-3 Clinical grades given by faculty and resident raters and examination scores for 36 medical students.

bitious purposes than simply addressing the strength of the associations. Regression techniques can provide details about the association. As patients gain weight, systolic blood pressure rises. But how much? If all our patients gained 10 kg, how much would the average blood pressure rise? Or, more importantly, if each of our overweight patients lost 10 or 20 kg, what kind of a reduction in blood pressure might we expect? Simple correlation coefficients are unit-free; that is, they measure the strength of a relationship but do not describe the magnitude of change among variables. Regression models do this. For every kilogram that body weight changes, systolic pressure changes 0.4 mmHg, on average.

Regression techniques are being seen increasingly in medical journals as methods of describing diagnostic and therapeutic predictive models.[4] Regression models can sort through groups of variables and consider the role of a number of factors simultaneously in predicting clinical outcomes. Which items of history and physical exam contribute most to predicting the patients with sore throat who will have streptococcal pharyngitis?[5] What clinical and laboratory information best identifies patients at risk for deep venous thrombosis after major abdominal surgery?[6] What groups of symptoms and electrocardiographic findings best discriminate chest-pain patients who have myocardial ischemia from those with noncardiac pain?[7] Regression models can evaluate a number of potential predictors, such as fever, tonsillar exudates, tender cervical nodes, antithrombin III concentration, substernal location of pain, and ST-segment depression to determine which contribute significantly to identifying patients who have streptococcal pharyngitis, are at risk of deep venous thrombosis, or need admission to the coronary care unit. They can also tell us the relative amount or weight each variable contributes to predicting the outcome of interest.

There are a number of variations on the regression theme. A reader will encounter intimidating terms such as "logistic regression," "discriminate function analysis," "log linear models," and "stepwise multiple regression." These are all forms of regression procedures that involve manipulating multiple variables simultaneously to determine which best predicts the outcome.

An example of this useful technique is found in a paper by Slap and co-workers,[8] who studied the question of when to perform biopsies of enlarged peripheral lymph nodes. Faced with the adolescent or young adult with peripheral lymphadenopathy, when does the clinician recommend a biopsy to assess the risk of serious disease? If the enlarged node is "benign" and requires no treatment, one would like to avoid the expense and discomfort of biopsy. If there is a substantial risk of treatable disease such as tuberculosis or malignancy, a biopsy is most useful.

Slap and colleagues analyzed the charts of 123 patients who had enlarged peripheral nodes. For each of these patients there was a histopathological diagnosis that the authors classified into one of two categories, "no treatment" or "treatment." Either the biopsy was "normal," showed "reactive hyperplasia," or was otherwise indicative of a nontreatable condition or showed evidence of granulomatous reaction or malignancy and suggested that therapy was needed.

The authors reviewed 22 clinical variables for each of the patients, including demographic features; site of the node(s); signs and symptoms such as fever, night sweats, weight loss, and other organ enlargement; and results of several laboratory investigations. Each variable was first assessed for possible association with the "treatment" or "no treatment" outcome using the chi-square test. Clinical factors that appeared to be related to the outcome—that is, that had a statistical association ($p < .01$)—were entered into a stepwise discriminate analysis program. This statistical model considers each of the variables in relation to one another and develops a linear equation using only the variables that best predict whether a patient's lymph node is in the treatment or no-treatment category. Of the 22 clinical variables considered, only 3 were found to make independent contributions to predicting the need for treatment. If a lymph node was greater than 2 cm in size or the chest roentgenogram was abnormal, the node was more likely to require treatment. If the patient had a recent history of ear, nose, and throat symptoms such as earache, coryza, or sore throat, the enlarged node was less likely to require treatment.

Using the findings of their discriminate function model, the authors were able to correctly classify 95 percent of their lymphadenopathy patients who required treatment and correctly classify 96 percent of their no-treatment group. In the next chapter we will discuss in more detail how they translated their statistical model into a clinical decision-making tool.

Regression models add more statistical nomenclature to the reader's vocabulary. Each variable that contributes to the predictive model will have its own *coefficient*. This may be a positive or negative number and simply indicates the weighting the variable has in the model. For the scatterplot depicting the relationship between weight and systolic blood pressure, the regression equation BP = 99 + .45 (weight in kilograms) describes the relationship mathematically (Fig. 9-4). The general form of this equation is $y = a + bx$, where a is the theoretical point of intercept on the y axis when x is equal to zero, and b is the amount of change in the y variable for every unit change of x. Practically speaking, this means that we can predict, on average, our patients' systolic blood pressures from their weights. Starting with 99 mmHg of pressure, we add 0.45 times weight to derive systolic pressure. In other words, for every additional kilogram of weight, blood pressure increases almost 0.50 mm. Remember, of course, that the equation is simply our best summary estimate of the blood pressure–weight relationship and that individual patient values will vary from the model just as they do in the scatterplot.

A term that is often used in describing correlation and regression relationships is r^2. r^2 is the square of the correlation coefficient r. It is

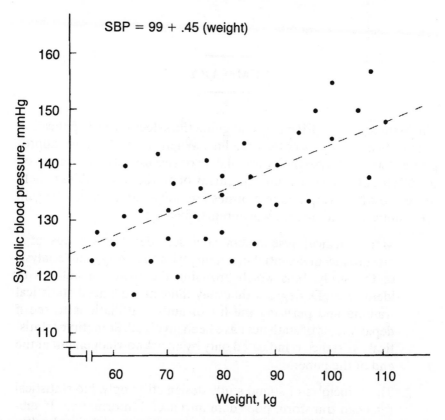

FIGURE 9-4 Systolic blood pressure (SBP) and weight of 36 patients.

interpreted as representing the amount of variance in an outcome variable (such as blood pressure) that can be attributed to changes in a predictor variable (such as weight). In our example, the correlation coefficient r was .69. Squaring r, we obtain a value of .48, which we can interpret as indicating that 48 percent of the variance in the patient's blood pressure is due to weight. Stated another way, differences in weight predict almost half of the variability we observe in blood pressures. The remaining 52 percent is due to other factors.

This means that correlation coefficients must be relatively high (close to 1.0) before the association they describe can be said to "explain" a substantial proportion of the outcome. If we were to find, for example, that length of waiting time in the doctor's office correlates with patient satisfaction with $r = .3$, our results would indicate that only 9 percent ($.3^2$) of patient satisfaction has been explained by length of wait.

SUMMARY

Understanding the principles that guide the selection and application of statistical tests aids critical reading. When researchers use appropriate tests to analyze their ordinal data or successfully use regression models to sort through a confusing array of predictor variables to help us decide when lymph node biopsies are indicated, their results gain credibility. Several tips are worth remembering:

1. Many medical researchers now consider the services of a biostatistician essential in helping with the design and analysis of the study. It is worth browsing the roster of authors to identify Ph.D. degrees that may indicate advanced statistical training and perusing the list of author affiliations to see if departments of statistics have been involved. Sometimes statistical assistance is indicated only by an acknowledgement at the end of the paper.

2. The principles of sound study design still apply. No statistical tests can transform poor data into useful information. If subjects are unwittingly selected because they are sicker or health-

ier or more cooperative, if blood pressures are measured by a biased observer, or if there are differing levels of regimen compliance because Lydia Pinkham's Compound tastes better than Bull Durham's Extract, the most sophisticated regression model will not help.

3. A number of general-readership journals publish feature articles that review statistical topics. These are worth reading and saving as aids to critical review.

4. Statistical significance still does not mean clinical importance.

REFERENCES

1. Colton T: *Statistics in Medicine*. Boston, Little Brown, 1974.
2. Ingelfinger JA, Mosteller F, Thibodeau LA, Ware JH: *Biostatistics in Clinical Medicine*, 2nd ed. New York, Macmillan, 1987.
3. Moses LE, Emerson JD, Hosseini H: Analyzing data from ordered categories. *N Engl J Med* 311:442, 1984.
4. Godfrey K: Simple linear regression in medical research. *N Engl J Med* 313:1629, 1985.
5. Poses RM, Cebul RD, Collins M, Fager SS: The accuracy of experienced physicians' probability estimates for patients with sore throats: Implications for decision making. *JAMA* 254:925, 1985.
6. Sue-Ling HM, Johnston D, McMahon MJ et al: Pre-operative identification of patients at high risk of deep venous thrombosis after elective major abdominal surgery. *Lancet* 1:1173, 1986.
7. Pozen MW, D'Agostino RB, Selker HP, et al: A predictive instrument to improve coronary-care-unit admission practices in acute ischemic heart disease: A prospective multicenter clinical trial. *N Engl J Med* 310:1273, 1984.
8. Slap GB, Brooks JSJ, Schwartz JS: When to perform biopsies of enlarged peripheral lymph nodes in young patients. *JAMA* 252:1321, 1984.

CHAPTER TEN

INTERPRETATION: SENSITIVITY, SPECIFICITY, AND PREDICTIVE VALUE

Ford has a better idea.

WELL-KNOWN ADVERTISING SLOGAN

We live with a surfeit of other people's good ideas. The mail brings almost daily suggestions for enriching our medical knowledge while we are cruising through Caribbean islands or skiing in the Wasatch Mountains. Journals offer multi-colored proposals from pharmaceutical companies for reducing patient blood pressures or relieving contact dermatitis—mixed in with the latest epidemiologic pronouncements on the causes of endometrial cancer. Suggestions for improving our diagnostic capabilities also abound. Descriptive studies and cross-sectional designs touting clinical signs and symptoms, laboratory determinations, and radiographic procedures as aids in clinical decision making are much in vogue. Computed tomography and ultrasound devices claim to localize lacunae in our heads, holes in our hearts, and cysts in our kidneys. Old techniques such as the Gram stain and the C-reactive protein are revitalized and used to diagnose streptococcal pharyngitis. Clinical signs and symptoms are combined in different ways in an effort to best predict when stool cultures are likely to yield enteric pathogens. With all the new and not-so-new technological approaches available, it is difficult to decide which dishes among the diagnostic smorgasbord are most worthwhile. In this chapter, we will devote ourselves to interpreting evaluations of these diagnostic ideas and prediction tools.

There are several approaches to assigning value to a new test or clinical complex. The first, which is encountered with distressing frequency, is the author's proclamation that it is so. "In my experience, right upper quadrant pain means cholecystitis." "We have found that bilateral infiltrates on chest radiographs signify Legionnaire's disease." The presence of gallbladder disease in 8 out of 10 patients with abdominal pain, or the observation that the last five patients with chest films that had patchy infiltrates had antibody titers to *Legionella* are "swallows that do not a summer make." Uncontrolled observations filter into the most respected of publications. They may be useful as preliminary, descriptive hunches but should be challenged to provide evidence of validity and generalizability. "Author" and "authority" come from common Middle English stock and run the danger of becoming synonyms in the minds of some.

A somewhat more satisfactory approach to assessing a new diagnostic technique is to employ a statistical test of association to see if the new method helps discover disease more often than might be expected by chance. The article on blood culturing and bacteremia[1] relies on *p* values and statistical significance to support its claims for diagnostic effectiveness. Recall that one of the tidbits of information imparted from this study was that certain clinical and laboratory features were useful predictors of which children would ultimately be found to have bacteremia. Among these were age, fever, and white blood cell (WBC) count (see Table 10-1).

> Bacteremia was most frequent in children seven to twelve months old ($p < 0.001$) and was associated with a white cell count of 20,000 or more ($p < 0.01$) and a temperature of 39.4°C or higher ($p < 0.01$)[1]

Shunning the seduction of the small *p* value and remembering that statistically significant predictors may not be clinically useful guides, we find that Table 10-1 provides some helpful information. The frequency of positive blood cultures does rise with temperature as well as with WBC count and is higher in one of the younger age groups. It also appears that this observation is unlikely to be due to chance. But somehow we are not getting the complete picture. We know something of how valuable the fever and WBC count are in predicting disease

• TABLE 10-1 •

Factors associated with bacteremia in febrile pediatric outpatients

Factor	Positive cultures	Total cultures	Percent positive
Age (months)			
6 or less	1	74	1.4
7 to 12	11	116	9.5
13 to 24	5	131	3.8
25 or greater	5	225	2.2
Temperature (°C)			
Less than 38.9	2	159	1.3
38.9 to 39.4	4	99	4.0
39.4 to 39.9 (sic)	10	124	8.1
40.0 or higher	6	96	6.3
White blood cell count ($\times 10^3/mm^3$)			
Less than 10.0	2	162	1.2
10.0 to 19.9	13	193	6.7
20.0 or more	6	52	11.5

Source: Based on data from McGowan et al.[1]

when they are elevated: About 12 percent of the time, a high WBC count will identify a patient with bacteremia; 7 percent of the time, a temperature of 39.4°C or higher will accurately predict the problem. It is also clear, however, that these tests are not always right; they are correct only 12 and 7 percent of the time. That means that 88 of 100 and 93 of 100 times a high WBC count and a high fever incorrectly suggest that patients have bacteremia. Furthermore, the tests also fail to detect some patients who have disease. Not every patient who is bacteremic meets the criterion of temperature greater than 39.4°C or WBC count above 20,000/mm³. These are important errors in classification and are limitations in the tests that clinicians must incorporate into decision making. Pronouncements of statistical significance alone do not provide sufficient information.

Recasting some of the data contained in Table 10-1 into the schematic seen in Table 10-2 provides us with a better sense of how the tests are performing. A fever of 39.4°C or greater occurs in 220 of 478 patients. Sixteen of these children turn out to have bacteremia, for a frequency of about 7 percent. However, we can see from the table that 6 children who have positive blood cultures have temperatures

· TABLE 10-2 ·								
Factors associated with bacteremia in febrile pediatric outpatients								
	Temperature, °C (temp)				White blood cells/mm³ (WBC)			
		Blood culture				Blood culture		
		Positive	Negative	Total		Positive	Negative	Total
Temp	≥39.4°	16	204	220	WBC	≥20,000 6	46	52
	<39.4°	6	252	258		<20,000 15	340	355
		22	456	478		21	386	407

SOURCE: Based on data from McGowan et al.[1]

below 39.4°C. These children will be misclassified by the criterion of high fever. It is also apparent from inspecting the tables that while 252 of the 456 children who did not have bacteremia are correctly classified by the criterion of temperature below 39.4°C, a substantial number, 204, are incorrectly labeled as bacteremic. Similarly, a WBC count above 20,000/mm³ is an accurate predictor of bacteremia on 6 of 52 occasions, or 12 percent of the time. This test is much more accurate in identifying truly negative patients. In all, 340 of 386 children with negative blood cultures are appropriately classified by virtue of their low WBC counts. Only 46 children with negative blood cultures fall into the high-WBC group and are incorrectly called bacteremic. This is a much better batting average than the temperature criterion offered. Unfortunately, the WBC count misses more cases of bacteremia than it identifies. Only 6 of 21 positive cultures have concurrent WBC counts above 20,000/mm³; 15 bacteremia patients have WBC counts that fall below the cutoff point.

We have just described a systematic approach to evaluating diagnostic tests. Concepts known as *sensitivity*, *specificity*, and *predictive value*, terms familiar to many medical readers, are used to summarize the system.[2] As with other bits of jargon, a moderate amount of confusion has surrounded the application of these terms. Twenty house officers, 20 fourth-year medical students, and 20 attending physicians at four teaching hospitals were asked in "hallway encounters" to solve a medical problem that required calculating the predictive value of a test.[3] Only 11 of the 60 participants were able to come up with the correct answer. The reasoning is straightforward in the sensitivity, specificity, and predictive-value game, but it takes a bit of thought to digest the principles and—for most of us—a pencil and piece of paper for sketching a hasty two-by-two table like the one shown in Table 10-3.

Sensitivity is the ability of a test to single out people who have disease. For those who thrive on equations, using the notations in Table 10-3, sensitivity is $A/(A + C)$. *Specificity* is the ability of the test to classify people who do not have illness as negative. In the algebra of Table 10-3, it is $D/(B + D)$. The predictive value of a diagnostic endeavor gives the frequency with which a positive test actually signifies disease. Reading horizontally across Table 10-3, it is $A/(A + B)$. *Predictive value* is more properly designated as *positive* predictive value (the value of a positive test). Its companion, *negative* predictive value—the frequency with which a negative test identifies people without disease—is substantially less useful. Most authors are speaking positively when they refer to predictive value.

Let us return to the bacteremia data and attach some terms to the information we compiled. Table 10-4 summarizes the sensitivity, specificity, and predictive value for temperature and WBC count as diagnostic tests for bacteremia. The two tests may be compared, and the intuitive reservations we developed from examining Table 10-2 can be quantified. Using temperature to diagnose bacteremia, we will properly identify 73 percent of patients who have positive cultures. That is the sensitivity. Our specificity is not very high; only 55 percent of patients who are without disease will be properly identified by their position in the lower-temperature group. The predictive value of fever is low; only 7 percent of all children with temperatures above 39.4°C

• TABLE 10-3 •
Sensitivity, specificity, and predictive value

		Disease		
		Present	Absent	
Test	Positive	A	B	$A + B$
	Negative	C	D	$C + D$
		$A + C$	$B + D$	$A + B + C + D$

Sensitivity	$= A/(A + C)$
Specificity	$= D/(B + D)$
Predictive value	$= A/(A + B)$

• TABLE 10-4 •
Sensitivity, specificity, and predictive value of temperature and WBC count in diagnosing bacteremia

		Temperature, °C (temp)				White blood cells/mm^3 (WBC)			
		Blood culture					Blood culture		
		Positive	Negative	Total			Positive	Negative	Total
Temp	≥39.4°	16	204	220	WBC	≥20,000	6	46	52
	<39.4	6	252	258		<20,000	15	340	355
		22	456	478			21	386	407

Sensitivity	= 16/22 = 73%	Sensitivity	= 6/21 = 29%
Specificity	= 252/456 = 55%	Specificity	= 340/386 = 88%
Predictive value	= 16/220 = 7%	Predictive value	= 6/52 = 12%

SOURCE: Based on data from McGowan et al.[1]

will have positive blood cultures. The specificity of the WBC count, 88 percent, is much better. Sensitivity, however, suffers substantially when this test is used; only 29 percent of children with positive cultures are properly identified. The WBC count offers better predictive value: of the 52 children with elevated WBC counts, 12 percent have bacteremia.

There is a message in all this. Diagnostic tests are not perfect. Some degree of misclassification of patients is inevitable. By using attributes of sensitivity, specificity, and predictive value, we are able to quantify in a standard way the ability of any test to make correct and incorrect classifications. Some papers will speak of the efficiency of a test. *Efficiency* is an overall estimate of a test's ability to classify patients correctly. The boxes in Table 10-4 surround the numbers of patients who are correctly labeled. Efficiency is the combination of these two correct classification boxes divided by the total number of patients assessed. For temperature, this would be (16 + 252)/478, or 56 percent; for WBC count, the efficiency is (6 + 340)/407, or 85 percent.

The concept of efficiency may overly summarize the attributes of the test. White blood cell count appears to be a more efficient diagnostic test than temperature for detecting bacteremia. But how concerned is the clinician about missing cases of bacteremia? The high efficiency of WBC count is due largely to the fact that most patients have negative cultures and also have WBC counts below 20,000/mm^3. Over two-thirds of positive cultures are misidentified by using the criterion of the elevated WBC count. Sensitivity this low is not acceptable. If a disease is worth detecting, a 71 percent miss, or *false-negative*, rate is unacceptable. Elevated temperature is a more sensitive test; only about one-fourth of patients with positive cultures will fall into the false-negative category. On the other hand, when we choose fever, specificity suffers. Elevated temperatures were seen in 204 of the 456 patients with negative cultures. These are *false positives*, test results falsely indicating the presence of disease.

PREVALENCE

The purpose of a diagnostic test is to improve our level of certainty about the cause of a patient's illness. Sensitivity and specificity are useful gauges of a test's value. The higher these numbers, the better the test. But there are other factors to consider. The frequency or prevalence of the condition or disease in the population being tested is a major concern. Readers will encounter references to the pretest or prior probability and to posttest or posterior probability in discussions of diagnostic procedures. *Pretest*, or *prior, probability* is the prevalence of a condition in the study population. A pretest probability of 5 percent means that 5 of every 100 subjects in the total group being tested will have the condition. Thus our chances of correctly guessing the diagnosis *without* the benefit of diagnostic devices is 5 percent. *Posttest* or *posterior, probability* is the same as predictive value. We hope that after we know a test is positive, our ability to predict the presence of disease in that subgroup will be enhanced. Conversely, a negative test should result in a marked decrease in likelihood of disease from the pretest probability.

Table 10-5 shows the benefit of a positive diagnostic test that has a 90 percent sensitivity and 90 percent specificity for a disease with a pretest probability of 5 percent. The bottom row of the table indicates that 100 of every 2000 subjects tested (5 percent) have the disease in question (prevalence/pretest probability). Of those 2000 individuals, 280 will have a positive test (top row), and 90 of those who test positive

• TABLE 10-5 •

Prevalence/pretest probability and predictive value/posttest probability

		Disease		
		Present	Absent	
Test	Positive	90	190	280
	Negative	10	1710	1720
		100	1900	2000

Sensitivity	=90/100	=90%
Specificity	=1710/1900	=90%
Prevalence	=100/2000	= 5%
Predictive value	=90/280	=32%

will actually have disease. The ratio of 90/280 (32 percent) is the predictive value/posttest probability of a positive test and represents a sixfold improvement over the pretest level. The high sensitivity and specificity have worked to produce a test that substantially enhances diagnosis.

However, in some situations, where pretest probability/prevalence is very low, the value of tests with even high sensitivity and specificity may be reduced. Policies proposed by state legislatures to require mandatory premarital serological testing for HIV prompted researchers from Boston to estimate the benefits of a premarital screening program.[4] Initial screening was to be done with an enzyme immunoassay (EIA) that the authors estimated had a sensitivity of 98.3 percent and a specificity of 99.8 percent. These are impressive numbers indeed. It is hard to find a more accurate test in any arsenal. The key to the analysis, however, is the estimate of the prevalence or pretest probability of HIV. As we saw in Chap. 4, these prevalence estimates vary widely. Since no data were available on the actual frequency of HIV among the premarital population, the authors used information derived from blood donors. The figure they came up with was only 35 positives for every 100,000 individuals tested. When test characteristics and this pretest probability are applied to the almost 4 million individuals who are married each year, the expected distribution of results is as seen in Table 10-6.

• TABLE 10-6 •

Expected enzyme immunoassay results in 1-year premarital screening program

	HIV Infection	No Infection	HIV Total
Positive	1,325	7,648	8,973
Negative	23	3,816,372	3,816,395
Total	1,348	3,824,020	3,825,368

Sensitivity	=1,325/1,348	=98.3%
Specificity	=3,816,372/3,824,020	=99.8%
Prevalence	=1,348/3,825,368	=.035%
Predictive value	=1,325/8,973	=14.8%

Source: Based on data from Cleary et al.[4]

Despite the high levels of sensitivity and specificity, the very low prevalence of HIV infection in the premarital population creates a posttest probability of only 15 percent. This means that for every 1300 individuals correctly diagnosed as HIV-infected, there are over 7600 false positives. That is a great many people who will be unnecessarily alarmed by the specter of HIV.

The authors employed a second stage to the screening and submit EIA-positive individuals to a confirming test, the Western blot. The Western blot also has excellent test characteristics, with a sensitivity of 92 percent and specificity of 95 percent. But even after this second round, over 380 people remained falsely classified as HIV-positive. There is an important message here. Prevalence or pretest probability is critical to any screening or case-finding exercise. One needs to identify subjects with as high a pretest probability as possible before testing begins. In the case of HIV testing, subjects in a general premarital population who lack identified risk factors for HIV infection are not reasonable candidates for screening.*

---

*Despite the concerns raised by the Boston study,[4] Illinois instituted premarital HIV testing. Results of the first 6 months of the program were reported, and the yield of positive tests was even less than estimated.[5] Only 8 of more than 70,000 marriage-license applicants were seropositive for a frequency of 11 per 100,000. The estimated cost of the program was $2.5 million, or about $312,000 for every positive applicant.

MAKING CHOICES

The game of diagnostics is one of trade-offs. When we attempt to improve the sensitivity of our procedures and detect everyone who has an illness, we become less selective. We fall back on the most common denominator, like fever, and include people who do not have the disease. We can become more restrictive by raising the specificity of the test and reducing the number of false-positive determinations. But then sensitivity is bound to suffer.

Nevertheless, choices between sensitivity and specificity must be made. How do we decide where to draw the line between positive and negative and between sensitivity and specificity? The answer is not a statistical one. It is a clinical and economic decision. What are the costs of misclassifying patients? When the consequences of missing a disease are crucial, as in the case of a curable cancer or treatable, life-threatening bacterial infection, sensitivity is paramount. We are willing to risk misclassifying a few people as positives, especially if other, more definitive diagnostic procedures are available to correct our initial mistakes.

Screening programs to detect phenylketonuria (PKU) among newborns attempt to be very sensitive. Failure to detect cases of this treatable genetic disease will result in permanent mental retardation and great personal and social cost. A percentage of false positives will occur in these screening programs, but repeat blood tests are readily available to reclassify these babies correctly.

If, on the other hand, the burden of creating false positives outweighs the advantages of capturing all cases of a disease, increasing specificity should be the goal. If exploratory surgery or invasive angiography is necessary to confirm a diagnosis, high specificity is desirable. An example of a clinical sign that is frequently encountered and should be specific is the heart murmur. While the heart murmur can be a reasonably sensitive diagnostic aid for detecting valvular heart disease (most people with bad valves have murmurs), there are many people who have murmurs and perfectly normal hearts (false positives). Substantial medical costs can be incurred if extensive cardiac evaluation is performed on every patient who has a murmur. Thousands of cardiograms, chest x-rays, and even catheterizations can be done to document the absence of heart disease in patients misclassified by the presence of a murmur. Bergman and Stamm have even written about the psychological effects that can occur when children with "innocent" heart murmurs are thought by parents to be suffering from heart disease.[6] Activities become restricted as children are put into undesirable sick roles by diagnostic misclassification.

Let us recap the basics covered thus far. We have seen that for assessing the diagnostic worth of tests, proclamations of highly statistically significant associations are not sufficient, and that *p* values may cover the page without telling us what we want to know. Clinicians need information on the extent to which diagnostic tests misclassify subjects. Characteristics like sensitivity, specificity, and predictive value are tools necessary to making clinical decisions. We can learn the probability that tests will miss cases of disease (false negatives) and how likely it is a positive result will occur in a patient who is free of disease (false positives). In predictive value, we have an estimate of the likelihood that given a positive test, a patient will, in fact, have the illness in question. We have seen that predictive value is at the mercy of prevalence. Even a small percentage of false positives becomes magnified when a disease is rare, which reduces the likelihood that a positive test signifies disease. We have seen that the sensitivity and specificity of tests can change as decision points are altered. In some cases, a test must be highly sensitive in order to identify all cases of illness, and specificity is sacrificed. In other instances, the costs of creating false positives are intolerable, and specificity must be preserved at the expense of sensitivity.

MULTIPLE TESTS

Evaluating the diagnostic properties of just one test requires serious contemplation to learn the concepts and terminology we have just described. But the process of diagnosis rarely relies on results of a single symptom, physical finding, or laboratory determination. We gather and process many findings in making a diagnosis. We really need to know how these findings work in concert to aid our decisions. What is the likelihood of Rocky Mountain spotted fever if fever, headache, and rash are all present? What if only fever and rash occur? How can we cope with the confusion of multiple, often interrelated variables?

The *multivariate regression techniques* discussed in Chap. 9 can help. The study on lymph node biopsy illustrates the application of mathematical models to improve diagnostic decisions.[7] Recall that Slap et al. collected data on 22 clinical variables from 123 patients with enlarged peripheral lymph nodes. They used a regression model to identify the findings that best classified patients as requiring or not requiring treatment. Three of the findings made significant independent contributions to their predictive model: lymph node size greater than 2 cm, abnormal chest roentgenogram, and recent ear, nose, or throat symptoms. Some authors would have stopped here, feeling that they had fulfilled their mission by narrowing the clinician's concern from 22 to 3 variables. But how does one use this information to arrive at a decision? Are the factors equally important? What if only two of three are present? Slap et al. used regression equation coefficients to assign a weight to each of the findings and produce a practical scoring system. Each patient began with a score of −2 points based on the regression model constant. Five points were added for an abnormal chest roentgenogram and 3 points if the node was bigger than 2 cm, but 3 points were subtracted if ear, nose, or throat symptoms were present. When this "discriminant score" was tallied for each patient who had been classed in the treatment or nontreatment group, the distribution of scores appeared as in Fig. 10-1. Most of the no-treatment group have scores of −2 or below; most patients in need of treatment are at 1 or above. However, the distributions of scores for treatment and nontreatment patients overlap. No matter which discriminant score one picks to guide the decision to biopsy, some misclassification occurs. If all patients with scores greater than 0 are classified as needing a biopsy, and all patients whose scores are 0 or less are not biopsied, 4 misclassifications occur among the 88 patient scores depicted in the figure. The discriminant score at which a biopsy is recommended could be lowered to −2 or above. This would include all cases who subsequently fall into the treatment group but would misclassify a large number of no-treatment patients.

In their article, Slap et al. constructed a curve that is useful for depicting the trade-offs that occur when one selects different cutoff points of a diagnostic variable to make decisions. The *receiver-operating characteristic (ROC) curve* in Fig. 10-2 shows sensitivity (true positives) on the y axis and $1 -$ specificity (false positives) on the x axis. As one chooses different scores as decision points, changes in the ratio of true positives and false positives become apparent. For exam-

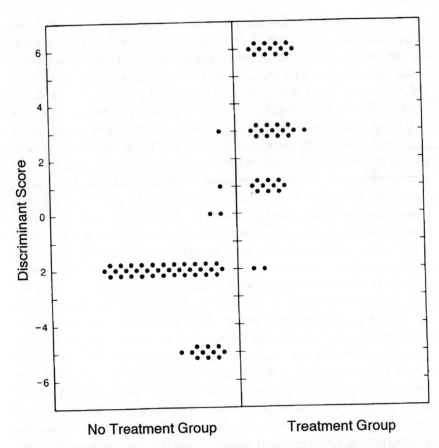

FIGURE 10-1 Discriminant scores of patients with peripheral lymphadenopathy whose biopsy results do not lead to treatment (no-treatment group) or do lead to treatment (treatment group). (From Slap et al.[7] Copyright 1984, American Medical Association. Reprinted by permission.)

ple, if we use point *B* on the curve, a discriminant score greater than 2, we will find a very low false-positive rate. Only 1 of 49 individuals in the no-treatment group is biopsied when 1 − specificity is only 2 percent. At the same time, sensitivity is not optimal. Of 39 patients who ought to be biopsied, 12 are not. From visual inspection of the ROC curve, the best discriminant point for this scoring system is obvious. It is point *C* in the upper left-hand corner of the graph. This point maximizes sensitivity while minimizing false positives. ROC curves can be constructed for any test in which data are continuous to assess the discriminating properties of the test. The quality of tests

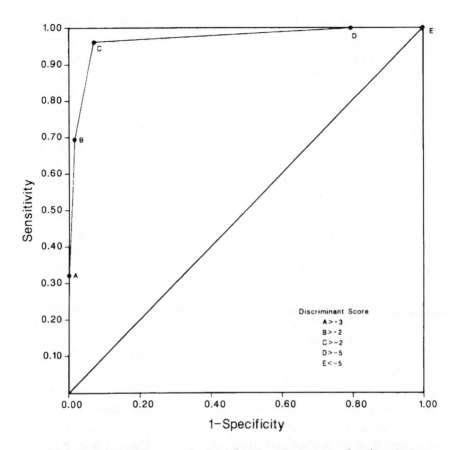

FIGURE 10-2 **Reviewer operating characteristic curve for discriminant scores of 88 patients at five cut points. Sensitivity = percentage of "treatment" cases correctly classified (true positives). 1–specificity= percentage of "no-treatment" cases incorrectly classified (false positives). (From Slap et al.[7] Copyright 1984, American Medical Association. Reprinted by permission.)**

may be assessed and compared using this methodology. The area that lies between the curve and the x axis can be estimated mathematically.[8,9] The more a curve arches into the upper left-hand corner, away from the nondiscriminatory diagonal (from 0 to E in Fig. 10-2), the greater the area beneath the curve and the better the test.

Many studies now use similar statistical approaches to create multivariate models for diagnostic and therapeutic decision making and for estimating patient prognosis. Modeling can help differentiate between bacterial and viral meningitis, guide treatment decisions for patients with pharyngitis, or predict the probability of mortality for patients admitted to intensive care units. In developing their mortality prediction model for such patients, Lemeshow et al. collected an array of information on 755 patients admitted to a combined medical/surgical intensive care unit.[10] Included were data on age, hospital service, blood pressure and pulse, presence of coma, infection, and cancer as well as a host of prior health conditions. The vital status of each patient at hospital discharge was also obtained. Each variable was assessed individually as a potential indicator of mortality. Those that were statistically significantly related to death or survival by a simple chi-square test became candidates for a multivariable logistic regression model. With many of the clinical variables—such as blood pressure and pulse rate—being interrelated, the statistical process helps to sort out the independent contribution of each factor and reduce the number of variables that are simply "along for the ride." Ultimately, only 7 of the 137 variables tested contributed to outcome prediction and were included in the model.

Models of this sort are useful. They help us marshal the multiple pieces of data we collect on our patients and combine them into a rational diagnostic or prognostic aid. But models have their limitations. Principles of population and sample selection still apply. When Poses et al. evaluated several prediction models for streptococcal pharyngitis, they explored how well the models could be "transported" from one clinical setting to another.[11] These decision aids were developed on data obtained from patients at a student health service and combined information on fever, pharyngeal exudate, cough, and cervical node tenderness to predict the presence of strep among patients with sore throats. In their original settings, the models performed well. However, the developmental data set came from a population where the prevalence of strep infection was 15 to 17 percent. Would the models perform as well in patient groups where the rate of streptococcal infection was lower? When the tests were applied to a new group of 310 subjects in whom the culture-proven prevalence of *Streptococcus* was only 5 percent, the models overestimated the frequency of streptococcal infection by as much as 93 percent.

The investigators postulated two possible explanations for this difficulty. Either the models had lost their discriminating power in the new patient population or the change in disease prevalence had altered the models' effectiveness.[11] To examine the former possibility, they compared ROC curve areas for the old and new study populations and found that the models performed their discriminating tasks well in both groups. This suggests that the change in prevalence had thrown predictions off kilter. Indeed, when the investigators adjusted their data statistically to match strep prevalence in the two populations, the models regained their predictive abilities. *Caveat emptor!* Even the most elegantly constructed, statistically sophisticated models travel from setting to setting at some peril.

SPECTRUM

Variations in the prevalence of a disease influence the utility of a test, but sensitivity and specificity may also vary, depending on the clinical stage of disease. A test that appears useful in an advanced state of illness may be less useful early in the disease course. Ransohoff and Feinstein refer to this as the problem of *spectrum*.[12] Diseases are dynamic and heterogeneous in nature and present a range of manifestations and bodily reactions as they progress. The interactions between host and disease differ in early stages of illness—colon cancer, rheumatoid arthritis, or bacterial endocarditis, for example—from those that occur later on. Tests that reflect the physiology or immune response of patients with overt, symptomatic illness may have little value in preclinical cases.

Documentation of the problem of spectrum and diagnostic test utility comes from the literature on screening tests for prostatic cancer. The authors of one study evaluated a radioimmunoassay for prostatic acid phosphatase in hopes that it would detect the disease early in its course, when treatment would be more effective.[13] Unfortunately, they found that the value of the test varied with the stage of progression of the cancer. In later stages of the disease, the test had reasonably high sensitivity. It identified between 71 and 92 percent of cancer patients. However, in the earlier stage I, only one-third of patients with known prostate cancer tested positive. The problem of spectrum is important. It has a surprisingly similar flavor to the whole business of population selection that has recurred so frequently throughout the book.

Screening for colorectal cancer with a carcinoembryonic antigen (CEA) offers another example.[14] This test is reasonably sensitive in finding advanced colorectal cancer of Duke's stages C or D at rates of

74 and 83 percent, respectively. However, detection at earlier stages, where treatment is likely to be more effective, is much less successful, with a sensitivity of only 36 percent.

Patient referral and selection patterns may also influence test characteristics. Researchers from Los Angeles were surprised by the apparent decline, over several years of use in their institution, in specificity of exercise radionuclide ventriculography as an aid to diagnosing coronary artery disease.[15] To clarify these impressions, they analyzed the results of ventriculography among 77 angiographically *normal* patients during two consecutive periods of time. Patients evaluated in the first 2-year period had a high proportion of normal responses (80 to 90 percent specificity) for the test. Patients evaluated during the later 3 years demonstrated normal responses only 35 to 50 percent of the time. One explanation for these results recalls the recurrent theme of selection bias. The investigators found that patients in the early group were a healthier sample than those tested later on. The subjects were younger, had less angina, and could endure bicycle exercise longer. When risk factors were combined, the pretest probability of coronary artery disease was five times higher for patients who were tested later. The sobering conclusion was that "sicker patients" will have a higher rate of abnormal ventriculography responses even though the "gold standard" of angiography is "normal." The authors also note a second factor that appeared to contribute to the declining specificity of the test. They found that confidence in the accuracy of radionuclide ventriculography had prompted clinicians to schedule the test *prior* to performance of angiography. Patients with abnormal ventriculography became preferentially selected for referral for angiograms during the late time period. Early on, angiography preceded ventriculography in most cases. Changes in test sequencing over time and consequent changes in the selection of patients who received both diagnostic procedures appeared to influence the assessment of the accuracy of ventriculography.

STANDARDS

To this point we have devoted our discussion to the diagnostic tests or clinical signs being evaluated, but we have paid little mind to the standards against which tests are compared. We have taken for granted that we really knew who had prostate cancer or bacteremia. How do we know who truly has disease and who does not? Are the standards against which we measure tests valid? The answer depends on which standard we use, since standards vary widely. Sometimes biopsy and histologic examination are utilized, other times serology; still other tests are validated by combinations of clinical impressions and laboratory or radiologic determinations. It should be remembered that all these methods have their own limitations and rates of error. Pathologists can misinterpret histological sections, serological tests may in themselves lack sufficient sensitivity to uniformly detect disease, and clinical impressions are woefully susceptible to observer error.

Familiar principles from previous chapters should rattle in our ears. Standards are diagnostic end points and—like entry criteria, treatment descriptions, and other determinations of outcome—must be clearly and satisfactorily defined. Biases can be introduced by observers who know of the test results before they read histologic sections or count colonies on the confirming culture. Conversely, knowledge of the true diagnosis may influence the interpretation of radiologic scans or findings on physical examination. Watch for these. Test results may affect the rigor with which standards are applied. When a test is positive, clinicians will look harder to find disease than when results are negative. More tests are ordered, additional x-rays are obtained, exploratory surgery is undertaken. Standards are unevenly applied. Often this cannot be avoided, since it is difficult to subject patients to invasive and expensive procedures without some justification.

Evaluations of screening programs for breast cancer are hampered by the uneven assessment of truth brought about by this workup bias. When techniques like mammography are assessed as screening tests for breast cancer, the standard is determined by biopsy. Women with suspicious lesions will have histologic diagnoses made. True positives and false positives can be reasonably estimated. We will have a good idea of the test's predictive value. Valid estimates of sensitivity will be much less satisfactory. Women for whom mammography is negative do not have breast biopsy to find malignancies unless some other tests hint at the presence of a lesion. Yet some undetected cancers are certain to exist. These will be false negatives that will go unappreciated because we are unable to apply our standard uniformly. Even when alternative tests turn up cancers that mammography fails to find, our best guess of sensitivity will remain an overestimate.

For many diseases, a single valid standard is not available. Take heart attack, for example. Without autopsy evidence of coronary occlusion and tissue death, the diagnosis of myocardial infarction must be made on a combination of clinical and laboratory features. Most clinicians rely on history of chest pain, evidence of disturbed myocardial rhythm or function, the results of the electrocardiogram, and a variety of serum-enzyme determinations to make the decision whether or not a patient has had a heart attack. While using a combination of clinical and laboratory observations is a perfectly legitimate diagnostic technique, it is not permissible to use the results of the test being evaluated as part of the standard. Surprisingly enough, this has been done. Studies have described the utility of particular muscle enzyme patterns in predicting myocardial infarction and have included, in the criteria for truth, clinical impressions that incorporate the enzyme results. It is not surprising to find reasonably good sensitivity for a test that is both predictor and standard.

COST CONSIDERATIONS

With the economic aspects of health care drawing increasing attention, it is not surprising that costs are becoming a concern in evaluations of diagnostic procedures and therapeutic interventions. Many articles that describe new diagnostic tests, clinical prediction devices, or alternative treatments try to balance the economic implications of benefits and adversities that might ensue. Included in the vocabulary of these assessments are terms such as *cost-benefit analysis, cost-effectiveness analysis*, and *sensitivity analysis.*

When Cebul and Poses evaluated predictive models for streptococcal pharyngitis, they considered not only the accuracy of their predictions but also the economic impact of treatment decisions that might result.[16] In constructing a cost-effectiveness analysis, they calculated the dollar value associated with correctly identifying and treating those pharyngitis patients with strep. A variety of components enter into the cost calculations. Items directly related to medical care are obviously important and include the costs of throat cultures and penicillin treatment. But there are many other costs to consider. Costs accrue when patients pay for office visits or are hospitalized for sequelae of the streptococcal infections or adverse reactions to treatment (e.g., penicillin allergy). In some analyses, nonmedical costs are included. These can extend to patient transportation expenses, time lost from work, and even the larger social costs of long-term disability and lost production. Many cost-effective analyses also include intangibles—such as quality-adjusted years of life, patient preferences, or utilities—when they calculate the value of a test or treatment. Would patients rather live 5 years longer with some disability or 3 years longer with none? The nuances become considerable and complex but are well explained for those who wish to know more.[17]

In Cebul's and Poses' analysis, costs are made up of the average cost of the medical evaluation and treatment, plus the costs associated with episodes of acute rheumatic fever that occur when some cases of strep are missed, plus the costs of treating side effects of therapy. The authors then compare four decision models against the actual performance of physicians who collected the data from sore-throat patients. Each of the prediction models proved more cost-effective than the physicians' actual practice. The best model was estimated to cost $32 for each correct decision, compared with $50 for each appropriate physician decision.

Many assumptions are necessary in economic analyses. One must estimate the frequencies of adverse health effects and drug reactions as well as a variety of medical costs. These components may vary depending on the season, region of the country, or patient population being served. To test the ability of their analysis to withstand variations in the underlying assumptions, Cebul and Poses performed a *sensitivity analysis*. They recalculated values using varying estimates of the frequency of rheumatic fever and allergic reactions to penicillin and the costs of throat cultures and other aspects of medical care. Do results differ if throat cultures cost $8 or $20, if the rate of rheumatic fever among untreated cases is 1 percent or 3 percent? The authors found that cost-effectiveness changed with the sensitivity analysis. Under certain assumptions, the best model cost only $20 for a correct decision. The highest cost was $74, variation in the cost of throat cultures being the most important determinant. Sensitivity analyses are helpful in interpreting exercises of this type. They allow readers to determine the robustness of the tests or models being evaluated—that is, their ability to withstand the variability that we know exists in the clinical world.

Sensitivity, specificity, and predictive value are tools clinicians can use to evaluate the cornucopia of diagnostic offerings described in medical journals. In the final analysis, the clinician must decide whether taking on a new test is beneficial. Clinical benefits must be weighed against medical risks and financial liabilities. Do blood cultures really improve the ability to identify seriously ill children? Do the costs of performing CT scans on patients with headaches pay off? Does the poor specificity of mammography, which results in biopsy of many women without malignant breast disease, negate its value as a diagnostic test? These are difficult questions, but it is essential that every new diagnostic test undergo rigorous scrutiny. If the test does not do it better or less expensively, it is not worth using.

SUMMARY

When articles offer information on new diagnostic tests, new applications of old tests, or novel ways of utilizing clinical symptoms and signs to identify diseases, ask the following:

1. Have sensitivity, specificity, and predictive value been calculated? Do the authors give evidence that they understand the importance of misclassifying patients into disease (false-positive) or nondisease (false-negative) categories? Has predictive value been correctly ascertained with reference to the prevalence of the disease in the population?

2. Has the problem of spectrum been considered? Do subjects on whom a test's sensitivity and specificity are being determined have severe or late-stage manifestations of disease? Are the results of tests on these individuals likely to apply to subjects who are less ill?

3. Is a reasonable standard being used? Are the histological-serological or clinical impressions being used to measure the test's validity reasonable proxies of truth? Have standards been applied equally to all patients in the evaluation? If not everyone has had an x-ray or blood test, have patients who truly have disease been missed? Have authors avoided the temptation to

include the test being evaluated as part of the standard? Have they guarded against bias by keeping standard evaluators protected from the influence of knowing test results?

4. Does the test improve on the present state of affairs? Is it more accurate, less costly, less painful, less time consuming, or in some other way better than the diagnostic techniques currently in practice?

REFERENCES

1. McGowan JE Jr, Bratton L, Klein JO, Finland M: Bacteremia in febrile children seen in a "walk-in" pediatric clinic. *N Engl J Med* 288:1309, 1973.
2. Sox HC: Probability theory in the use of diagnostic tests: An introduction to critical study of the literature. *Ann Intern Med* 104:60, 1986.
3. Casscells W, Schoenberger A, Graboys TB: Interpretation by physicians of clinical laboratory results. *N Engl J Med* 299:999, 1978.
4. Cleary PD, Barry MJ, Mayer KH, et al: Compulsory premarital screening for the human immunodeficiency virus: Technical and public health considerations. *JAMA* 258:1757, 1987.
5. Turnock BJ, Kelly CJ: Mandatory premarital testing for human immunodeficiency virus. *JAMA* 261:3415, 1989.
6. Bergman AB, Stamm SJ: The morbidity of cardiac non-disease in schoolchildren. *N Engl J Med* 276:1008, 1967.
7. Slap GB, Brooks JSJ, Schwartz JS: When to perform biopsies of enlarged peripheral lymph nodes in young patients. *JAMA* 252:1321, 1984.
8. Hanley JA, McNeil BJ: The meaning and use of the area under a receiver operating characteristic (ROC) curve. *Diagn Radiol* 143:29, 1982.
9. Swets JA: Measuring the accuracy of diagnostic systems. *Science* 240:1285, 1988.
10. Lemeshow S, Teres D, Pastides H, et al: A method for predicting survival and mortality of ICU patients using objectively derived weights. *Crit Care Med* 13:519, 1985.
11. Poses RM, Cebul RD, Collins M, Fager SS: The importance of disease prevalence in transporting clinical prediction rules. *Ann Intern Med* 105:586, 1986.
12. Ransohoff DF, Feinstein AR: Problems of spectrum and bias in evaluating the efficacy of diagnostic tests. *N Engl J Med* 299:926, 1978.
13. Foti AG, Cooper JF, Herschmyan H, Malvaex RR: Detection of pros-

tatic cancer by solid-phase radioimmunoassay of serum prostatic acid phosphatase. *N Engl J Med* 297:1357, 1977.

14. Fletcher RH: Carcinoembryonic antigen. *Ann Intern Med* 104:66, 1986.
15. Rozanski A, Diamond GA, Berman D, et al: The declining specificity of exercise radionuclide ventriculography. *N Engl J Med* 309:518, 1983.
16. Cebul RD, Poses RM: The comparative cost-effectiveness of statistical decision rules and experienced physicians in pharyngitis management. *JAMA* 256:3353, 1986.
17. Eisenberg JM: Clinical economics: A guide to the economic analysis of clinical practices *JAMA* 262:2879, 1989.

CHAPTER ELEVEN

INTERPRETATION: RISK

Beware the Jabberwock, my son!
The jaws that bite, the claws that catch!
Beware the Jubjub bird, and shun
The frumious Bandersnatch!

LEWIS CARROLL, Through the Looking Glass

*R*isks lurk everywhere. If you have bronchitis, inhaling pollutants puts you at risk of exacerbation. Placing a foot down on the accelerator pedal of your Porsche increases your risk of automotive mortality. Consuming nitrite preservatives and food dyes may predispose you to cancer. Simply belonging to a family in which heart disease or diabetes prevails can increase your chances of developing these diseases later in life.

Clinicians are faced with scores of implicit risks each day. They must constantly balance the benefits of treatment plans against potential liabilities. How likely is a 21-year-old primigravida with elevated blood pressure and proteinuria to develop eclampsia at delivery? What is the probability that a child with a febrile convulsion will develop epilepsy? What do you tell a 49-year-old with gallbladder disease about chances of surviving a cholecystectomy? Although the numbers are not always there to quantify the choices, the use of risk to weigh therapeutic choices and estimate future events occurs constantly in the clinical setting.

Risk serves several additional purposes in journal articles. Researchers use comparative risks to unravel the etiology of diseases, such as toxic-shock syndrome and breast cancer, or to demonstrate the effectiveness of interventions such as vaccination or isoniazid prophylaxis in preventing polio and tuberculosis. Public health planners gauge the risks of sexually transmitted diseases or drug abuse among subgroups of our population in order to focus their intervention efforts.

In this chapter we will examine the concept of risk as it is presented in medical journals and try to make a potential Jabberwock less intimidating.

STATEMENTS OF RISK

Basic risk statements express the likelihood that a particular event will occur within a particular population—for example, the number of cases of aplastic anemia among patients taking chloramphenicol or the frequency with which Down syndrome will occur in babies born to women over 40 years old. The virtue of the basic risk statement lies with its denominator: the number of people at risk. All too often when we read of medical events, we learn only of the numerator—that is, of the patients who developed aplastic anemia or who came down with toxic-shock syndrome. Knowing the denominator helps. Despite the adverse publicity directed at chloramphenicol, aplastic anemia occurs only once in every 30,000 to 40,000 doses.[1] Notwithstanding the flurry of controversy surrounding toxic-shock syndrome and tampon use, the risk of developing the disease is on the order of only 6 cases for every 100,000 menstruating women per year.[2] Risks are proportions that keep medical adversities in their place.

Not surprisingly, our best estimates of risk come from follow-up studies that observe cohorts of people and monitor their outcomes. Natural history studies that watch for the frequency of renal complications in schoolgirls with bacteriuria or the development of postpartum depression among women who have lost infants offer estimates of risk that provide valuable guides for prognosis and management.

RELATIVE RISK

Much that is published in medical journals concerns not simply the natural history of things but the quest for explanations. What are the causes of disease, and what steps can modern medicine take to reduce the likelihood of disability and death? In the search for etiology, there are specific ways of defining and comparing risks. Readers will encounter terms such as "relative risk," "relative odds," "risk ratio," and "odds ratio" as descriptors that attempt to get at the causes of disease. The relative risk compares the likelihood that a disease or outcome will occur among individuals who have a particular characteristic, exposure, or risk factor with the likelihood that the outcome will occur in individuals who do not have it. The higher the ratio, the stronger the association between the factor and the disease. Let us consider some examples.

The search for causes of coronary artery disease has been a medical obsession for some years. A host of factors ranging from eating, drinking, and smoking habits to blood pressure and cholesterol levels to genetic attributes have been examined in an attempt to increase our understanding of the disease. Among the more interesting studies are those demonstrating increased risk of heart disease among men who exhibit certain personality characteristics. A so-called coronary-prone behavior pattern, or type A personality, has been characterized by

> competitiveness, striving for achievement, aggressiveness, time urgency, restlessness, hyperalertness, explosiveness of speech amplitude, tenseness of facial musculature and feelings of struggle against the limitations of time and insensitivity of the environment. This torrent of life is usually, but not always, channeled into a vocation or profession with such dedication that type-A persons often neglect other aspects of their life such as family and recreation.[3]

In a follow-up study of 2700 men conducted in the mid-1960s[3] subjects completed questionnaires to provide information on the presence of these type A characteristics. Subjects were ranked by behavior scores and followed for four years to see who developed coronary artery disease. The annual risk of heart disease among men who exhibited the highest number of type A behavioral attributes was

14.3 per 1000, compared with 8.0 per 1000 for men with calmer behavior. Men with intermediate scores showed an intermediate rate. Comparing the risks for the highest and lowest scores, a relative risk of 14.3/1000 divided by 8/1000, or 1.8, is obtained. In other words, men exhibiting a high degree of type A behavior were almost twice as likely to develop heart disease during the follow-up period as men without these characteristics. Personality appears to have a role in causing heart disease.

Risk need not be viewed in negative terms. Other investigators who were looking for factors that would predict survival of patients who were discharged from a coronary care unit discovered that the support offered by "animal companions" provided protection from mortality.[4] Ninety-two men and women who were recovering from heart attacks or bouts of angina pectoris supplied information on a broad range of personal topics, including pet ownership. A year after hospitalization, follow-up was made to discover the status of the patients. Fourteen of the ninety-two had died. When death rates were calculated according to pet ownership, only 3 of 53 pet owners (5.6 percent) were no longer living, compared with 11 of 39 (28 percent) patients who were without animal companions. The relative risk of 5.6 per 100 divided by 28 per 100, or 0.2, means only one-fifth the mortality, or a fivefold greater likelihood of survival, if one has a furry or a feathered friend. That's an impressive difference! Perhaps prescriptions for dachshunds rather than digitalis should be offered at discharge from coronary care units.

RELATIVE RISK AND STUDY DESIGN

When we start with a population, as we do in follow-up studies, the calculation of relative risk is straightforward. We know in advance who eats carrots and who does not. We classify these people and remeasure them later to see who has developed poor eyesight. Table 11-1 illustrates how relative risk is created when a population with known risk-factor status is observed.

Case-control studies are trickier. Since the design enlists patients who already have poor vision, sorts them according to who consumes carrots, and makes the comparison with an independently selected control group, a common population base is lacking. The true risk of

	Disease present	Disease absent	
Factor present	A	B	$A + B$
Factor absent	C	D	$C + D$

• TABLE 11-1 •
Relative risk in population-based (follow-up) studies

Relative risk $= \dfrac{\text{rate of disease in people with factor}}{\text{rate of disease in people without factor}}$

$= \dfrac{\text{disease present/people with factor}}{\text{disease present/people without factor}}$

$= \dfrac{A/(A + B)}{C/(C + D)}$

Disease prevalence $= \dfrac{A + C}{A = B + C + D}$

disease cannot be calculated. We need to know about the relative rates of developing bad eyesight, not the relative rates of carrot eating. The problem is depicted in Table 11-2. We cannot move horizontally across the table to develop rates of disease for persons with and without a particular factor. The expression "$A/(A + B) / C/(C + D)$," which would give us the relative risk, cannot be calculated because the cases and controls are not represented in relation to their prevalence in any parent population.

However, there are ways of estimating relative risk from the case-control design. By tolerating two assumptions, we can come up with a serviceable substitute. First, we must hope that the control group is reasonably representative of the general population with respect to the occurrence of risk factors. Then, if the disease is relatively uncommon (as is true with most noninfectious diseases), A and C in Table 11-2 will be quite small in comparison with B and D. If we simply use B and D as approximations for $A + B$ and $C + D$,

---

• **TABLE 11-2** •

Relative risk estimate in case-control studies

	Cases	Controls	
Factor present	A	B	$A + B$
Factor absent	C	D	$C + D$

Relative	$=$	$\dfrac{\text{rate of disease in people with factor}}{\text{rate of disease in people without factor}}$
But ...		$\dfrac{A}{A+B}$ and $\dfrac{C}{C+D}$ do not represent rates of disease in a population
If ...		disease has a low frequency, so that A and C are small relative to B and D in the population at large
Then ...		$\dfrac{A}{B}$ approximates $\dfrac{A}{A+B}$
		and
		$\dfrac{C}{D}$ approximates $\dfrac{C}{C+D}$
And ...		relative risk is approximated by $\dfrac{A/B}{C/D}$ or $\dfrac{A \times D}{B \times C}$

---

respectively, the problem of disease frequency no longer interferes with our calculations. The estimate of relative risk can be expressed as A/B / C/D or, in simplified form, AD/BC. This cross-product estimate of relative risk is referred to as the *relative odds*, or *odds ratio*. Epidemiological purists are careful not to call this calculation a true relative risk, since the individual risk rates are approximations only.

Multiple sclerosis is an example of an uncommon disease, of uncertain etiology, that occurs with a frequency ranging from 10 to 100 cases per 100,000 population. One of many hypotheses put forth to explain this mysterious illness has been the accidental infection of man with viruses that normally reside in lower animals. One study conducted in Vermont sent postcard questionnaires to 100 patients with multiple sclerosis and 135 control subjects asking for information about contact with a variety of domestic animals and household pets.[5] A summary of the findings can be seen in Table 11-3. The increased

• **TABLE 11-3** •

Comparison of multiple sclerosis and control groups with respect to reported exposure to animal

Animals	Exposure to animals, %		
	Multiple sclerosis ($n = 100$)	Controls ($n = 135$)	Estimated odds ratio
Cats	65	57	1.4
Dogs	69	70	1.0
Rabbits	22	15	1.6
Horses	32	22	1.7
Cows	40	19	2.9
Chickens	37	14	3.6

SOURCE: Modified from Sylwester and Poser.[5]

frequency of exposure to animals for multiple sclerosis patients compared with controls creates odds ratios between 1 and 2 for cats, dogs, horses, and rabbits and larger risk estimates for contact with cows and chickens. Exposure to animals appears to be related to contracting multiple sclerosis. Detailed calculation of the odds ratio for chickens by the cross-product technique is shown in Table 11-4.

In another study on the same subject, Cook et al. demonstrated an association between contact with pet dogs and the development of multiple sclerosis.[6] Their analysis demonstrates another commonly

• **TABLE 11-4** •

Comparison of multiple sclerosis and control groups with respect to reported exposure to chickens

Exposed to chickens	Multiple sclerosis cases ($n = 100$)	Controls ($n = 135$)
Yes	37	19
No	63	116

$$\text{Odds ratio} = \frac{A \times D}{B \times C} = \frac{37 \times 116}{19 \times 63} = 3.6$$

SOURCE: Based on data from Sylwester and Poser.[5]

employed method of calculating risk ratios from case-control studies. In this study, for each patient diagnosed as having multiple sclerosis, a specific control subject was chosen who was matched by age, sex, race, and neighborhood of residence prior to the onset of symptoms in the subject. When this kind of careful matching is performed, a matched-pair analysis can be performed to calculate the odds ratio. The technique, as shown in Table 11-5, involves categorizing each case-control pair by concordance or discordance with respect to the characteristic under study. In the present example, 27 multiple sclerosis patients and their matched controls owned "indoor dogs"; four other pairs were also concordant in that neither case nor control reported dog ownership. Concordance, it turns out, tells us very little. The odds ratio for matched pairs is computed by comparing discordant categories. For 12 pairs of subjects, multiple sclerosis cases reported dog ownership when controls did not, compared with only 2 pairs in which controls were exposed to dogs and multiple sclerosis cases were not. The odds ratio can be directly computed as the ratio of these discordant groups, 12 / 2 or 6. In other words, ownership of a dog carries a sixfold risk of multiple sclerosis.

Recalling earlier discussions of sampling and inference, it should be clear that odds ratios determined from case-control studies are based on limited samples and are subject to sampling error. Knowl-

---

· TABLE 11-5 ·

Indoor dog ownership for multiple sclerosis patients and controls

		Dog ownership for pairs	
		Control	
		Yes	No
Multiple sclerosis patients	Yes	27	12
	No	2	4

$$\text{Odds ratio} = \text{ratio of discordant pairs}$$
$$= \frac{12}{2}$$
$$= \frac{\text{case "yes," control no}}{\text{case "no," control "yes"}}$$
$$= 6$$

SOURCE: Based on data from Cook et al.[6]

edgeable investigators recognize that their data supply only a single estimate of the true relative odds or relative risk. On the basis of their particular findings, they can calculate a range in which the true estimate is likely to fall by constructing a confidence interval (CI) for the risk estimate similar to the CI we calculated to depict the range of differences in antibiotic cure rates for urinary tract infections in Chap. 8. If an odds ratio of 4.5 were found with a 95 percent CI of 2.2 to 7.8, the odds estimate would appear to be a twofold risk at a minimum. The important feature to look for in assessing the confidence interval is whether the boundaries include unity. An odds ratio of 1 means there is no association between the putative risk factor and disease— that no association exists between risk factors (dog ownership) and diseases (multiple sclerosis).

ATTRIBUTABLE RISK

Implicit in the process of identifying and defining risk factors is the hope that somehow, by modifying or eliminating risk, health can be improved. How many lives could be saved if seat belts were used more? How much would morbidity be reduced by bringing everyone's blood pressure under control? What impact do we have on the incidence of congenital birth defects with a national rubella immunization campaign? Comparison of risks is useful in assessing health-care prevention and treatment programs; but where causation is best suggested by ratios of risks, health impact is addressed by examining the differences in risk rates. The *attributable* risk tells us the difference in rates between people who smoke, have high blood pressure, or have susceptibility to rubella and those who do not. It indicates how much of the morbidity or mortality of a disease can be attributed to the risk factor. Attributable risk quantifies the contribution risk factors make in producing disease within a population. By comparing attributable risk for different factors, we can begin to arrange informed health-care priorities. Mortality data from the study of British doctors' smoking habits[7] demonstrate the difference between relative risk and attributable risk, as Table 11-6 shows. The relative risk of lung cancer due to smoking is much greater at 32 than is the relative risk of myocardial infarction among smokers, which is only 1.4. However, heart disease is much more common than lung cancer. So, even though the relative

	Death rate (per 100,000 population)	
· TABLE 11-6 ·		
	From lung cancer	From coronary disease
For heavy smokers	223	516
For nonsmokers	7	361
Relative risk	$\dfrac{223}{7} = 32$	$\dfrac{516}{361} = 1.4$
Attributable risk	$223 - 7 = 216$	$516 - 361 = 155$

· TABLE 11-6 ·
**Relative risk and attributable risk of cigarette smoking
for lung cancer and heart disease**

SOURCE: Based on data from Doll and Hill.[7]

risk associated with heart disease and smoking is small, its importance
to the general health is magnified. The death rate from heart disease
that can be attributed to smoking comes close to that contribued by
smoking-induced lung cancer. If cigarette smoking could be eliminated, almost as many deaths from coronary artery disease could be
prevented as from lung cancer.

BALANCING RISKS

The concept of risk helps quantify the likelihood of beneficial or
adverse medical outcomes and guides informed decision making, but
we can sometimes lose our perspective. Announcement that a new
environmental agent has been linked to cancer or that a drug may be
a risk factor for birth defects raises an emotional response that occasionally threatens rational decision making.

Because of the observation that women who smoke cigarettes
excrete reduced levels of estrogen in their urine and the known link
between estrogen and endometrial cancer, a case-control study was
conducted to determine whether cigarette smokers might have a
reduced incidence of this reproductive tract cancer.[8] A total of 510
women who had invasive endometrial cancer were interviewed for
historic information on use of a number of potential carcinogens. A

control group of 727 women who had other malignancies that are thought to be unrelated to cigarette use served as controls. Twenty-nine percent of controls were current smokers, compared with only 22 percent of endometrial cancer patients. The risk of cancer for smoking women was 0.7, with a 95 percent CI of 0.5 to 1.0. For women who smoked 25 cigarettes per day or more, the risk was even lower, at 0.5. This evidence suggests that smoking protects women from developing endometrial cancer, presumably by lowering estrogen secretion.

After all the terrible things we have said about cigarette smoking, here is evidence that the "evil weed" may have beneficial health effects. However, this "benefit" must be put into perspective with the overall adverse risk of tobacco use. The authors themselves are quick to point out that their results should not be interpreted as an endorsement for smoking. In an editorial commentary, Weiss[9] calculates that if smoking turned out to be protective, it would reduce the annual risk of endometrial cancer among postmenopausal women from approximately 100 per 100,000 to 70 per 100,000. On the basis of the mortality rate of the disease, he figures approximately 6 lives per 100,000 smokers would be saved annually. This is certainly not a large number and compares poorly with the lives *lost* annually because of cigarette smoking, which is estimated to be 30 times as high.[9]

Whenever medical decisions are made, adverse risks must be balanced against the potential benefits of the medication, surgical procedure, or immunization program. The controversy surrounding oral contraceptives is a case in point. Untoward effects of "the pill" have been a fertile ground for epidemiology researchers. A large number of papers have been published detailing possible associations between oral contraceptives and thromboembolic disease, stroke, heart attack, and high blood pressure. The publicity surrounding the controversy has made many physicians and patients shy away from the contraceptives. A summary editorial on the relationship between oral contraceptives and myocardial infarction suggested that women taking the pill were 2.5 to 5 times as likely to have a fatal heart attack as women not taking the pill.[10] This is a substantial increase in risk and gives reasonable cause for alarm. However, for women 30 to 39 years of age, this increased relative risk creates an absolute rate of only 3.5 deaths per 100,000 users per year. That is a very small number. An inquisitive reader might even ask if that tiny risk is not less than the risk of dying sometime in the course of pregnancy. That is an excellent question, and according to Morris,[11] British data suggest that the risk of dying from pregnancy is equal to or greater than that of dying from taking oral contraceptives.

In part, the perspective problem relates to limitations in basic study designs. Because complications from oral contraceptives are rare, most studies of associated morbidity and mortality are done in a case-control fashion. This means investigators can estimate the relative odds but do not have a population on which to base statements of absolute or attributable risk. We lack the denominators that are vital to determine rates of people at risk. For clinicians, it is an important omission.

Practicing doctors also need to know the risk tradeoffs in prescribing medication or advising surgery. What is the risk of anaphylaxis from penicillin given to treat strep throat compared with the risk of rheumatic fever if the patient goes untreated? Is the risk of death associated with gallbladder surgery offset by the benefits of the treatment? To make informed decisions, we must have comparable data about the gains as well as the liabilities of any course of action. The risks of all complications related to the use of oral contraceptives should be quantified and measured against the risks for other methods of birth control. These must then be balanced against the adverse outcomes associated with pregnancy. Data are not always available to quantify these risks. Frequently clinicians must make decisions based on insufficient information. It is important to remember, however, that when the adverse relative risk of a therapy is trumpeted by the news media, the magnitude of absolute risk and benefits of the treatment should also be considered.

SUMMARY

Statements of risk help us quantify the dangers of the environment; they serve as guides to prognosis and measures of potential effectiveness of health intervention activities. *Relative risk* is useful for testing hypotheses about etiologic association. *Attributable risk* provides a population perspective to assess the impact of changing risk factors on health.

Risk statements must be kept in perspective. Estimates of relative risk are derived from samples and, like any other samples, are vulnerable to error. Authors who place confidence intervals around their risk estimates provide readers with helpful information about the true likelihood that a factor is related to disease. Caution must be exercised in interpreting relative risk estimates without information about the absolute magnitude of risk. When risk factors are common, as with use of tampons or birth-control pills, and adverse outcomes such as toxic-shock syndrome or heart attack are uncommon, risks must be balanced against benefits. Before new treatments are advocated or established medications blacklisted, the overall health impact must be considered.

REFERENCES

1. Haile CA: Chloramphenicol toxicity. *South Med J* 70:479, 1977.
2. Davis JP, Chesney PJ, Wand PJ, et al: Toxic-shock syndrome: Epidemiologic features, recurrence, risk factors, and prevention. *N Engl J Med* 303:1429, 1980.
3. Jenkins CD, Rosenman RH, Zyzanski SJ: Prediction of clinical coronary heart disease by a test for the coronary-prone behavior pattern. *N Engl J Med* 290:1271, 1974.
4. Friedmann E, Katcher AH, Lynch JJ, Thomas SA: Animal companions and one-year survival after discharge from a coronary care unit. *Public Health Rep* 95:307, 1980.
5. Sylwester DL, Poser CM: The association of multiple sclerosis with domestic animals and household pets. *Ann Neurol* 2:207, 1979.
6. Cook SD, Natelson BH, Levin BE, et al: Further evidence of a possible association between house dogs and multiple sclerosis. *Ann Neurol* 3:141, 1978.
7. Doll R, Hill AB: Mortality in relation to smoking: Ten years' observations of British doctors. *Br Med J* 1:1399, 1460, 1964.
8. Lesko SM, Rosenberg L, Kaufman DW et al: Cigarette smoking and the risk of endometrial cancer. *N Engl J Med* 313:593, 1985.
9. Weiss NS: Can *not* smoking be hazardous to your health? *N Engl J Med* 313: 632, 1985.
10. Hennekens CH, MacMahon B: Oral contraceptives and myocardial infarction. *N Engl J Med* 296:1166, 1977.
11. Morris JN: *Uses of Epidemiology*, 3rd ed. Edinburgh, Churchill Livingstone, 1975.

CHAPTER TWELVE

INTERPRETATION: CAUSES

*...and now remains that we find out the cause of this effect.
Or rather say the cause of this defect. For this effect
defective comes by cause...*

Hamlet, Act II, Scene II

*P*oor Polonius, a tracker of truth, trapped in his own logical snares. He never does ferret out the cause of Hamlet's madness. Is it due to unrequited love, a father's death, or Denmark's melancholy climate? Polonius fails to find out. Indeed, he dies midway through the investigation, undone by his own hazardous techniques of study design.

Chasing after causes in medical studies is difficult though not usually terminal business. Up to now we have minced about with phrases such as "associated with," "linked to," and "related to." We have avoided dogmatic statements of causation, such as "Oral contraceptives cause vascular complications" or "Ingestion of lead paint is responsible for lower IQs among children." We have been reluctant to totally accept that vitamin C wards off colds or that birthing rooms are responsible for decreased problems in childbirth. Even when we think we have pinpointed the guilty party, the possibility remains that some unsuspected risk factor is actually causing the disease or an unappreciated cointervention is responsible for the treatment effect.

In this chapter, we will look for ways to decide whether the associations found in studies merit consideration as causes, and we will note some ways in which investigators deal with multiple potential explanations for the outcomes they observe.

CONFOUNDING

Spurious appearance of causation can occur through three mechanisms. The first of these is *chance*, where the caprice of sampling variability makes substance out of shadow. The rates of diarrhea caused by ampicillin and amoxicillin appear to be different but, in reality, sample estimates obtained from different portions of a single distribution of side effects create this illusion. We have considered all this in some detail in earlier chapters. *Bias* is the second mechanism. We have seen a variety of ways that spurious results may occur because our selection of comparison subjects is drawn from a sample of people with healthier lifestyles than case subjects or because the stress of illness has caused case subjects to recall their past medical history differently from controls. *Confounding* is the third mechanism.

In Chap. 3, we mentioned confusing or confounding factors in case-control studies. Confounding occurred when factors that related to both the characteristic under scrutiny and the outcome appeared as competing explanations. The example we used was the apparent etiological relationship between cigar smoking and baldness—an association that was confused or confounded by age. The data from this study appear in Table 12-1. We select 50 bald men to represent the cases and find that over one-half of them are cigar smokers. In the control group, only 8 of 50 subjects chosen admit to the habit. Using the cross-product estimation for the odds ratio, we see that there is a sixfold $[(27 \times 42)/(23 \times 8) = 1134/184 = 6.2]$ risk of baldness associated with cigar smoking. However, in examining the data, we realize that the ages of men in the groups being compared are dissimilar. Our bald subjects average 52 years of age, compared with a mean age of 24 years for controls. Quite a disparity! Since we know that increasing age is related both to cigar smoking and to loss of hair, we have a problem with confounding. Matching on age—that is, selecting only control subjects whose age is within several years of the case—is one

• TABLE 12-1 •

**Rate of cigar smoking for bald men compared
with controls**

		Baldness		
		Yes (cases)	No (controls)	
Cigar smoking	Yes	27	8	
	No	23	42	
		50	50	100

$$\text{Relative odds} = \frac{27 \times 42}{23 \times 8} = \frac{1134}{184} = 6.2$$

way of *controlling* the effects of age. When we redo our experiment, choosing only cases and controls who are between the ages of 40 and 45 years, the hypothetical results appear as in Table 12-2. Now the rates of cigar smoking are similar for cases and controls—that is, about 40 percent. The risk ratio, as calculated by the cross-products estimate, is very close to 1. There is no longer an association between smoking and hair loss. Confounding has been eliminated.

Confounding is the epidemiologist's eternal triangle. Any time a risk factor, patient characteristic, or intervention appears to be causing a disease, side effect, or outcome, the relationship needs to be chal-

• TABLE 12-2 •

**Rate of cigar smoking for bald men 40 to 45
years old compared with age-matched contorls**

		Baldness		
		Yes (cases)	No (controls)	
Cigar smoking	Yes	21	23	
	No	29	27	
		50	50	100

$$\text{Relative odds} = \frac{21 \times 27}{29 \times 23} = \frac{567}{667} = .85$$

lenged. Are we seeing cause and effect, or is a confounding factor exerting its unappreciated influence? The problem is schematized in Fig. 12-1. It is important to remember that to be a confounding variable, a factor must be related both to the outcome or effect and to the putative cause.

The apparent protective effect that animal companions afforded heart-attack victims[1] would seem to be a situation ripe for confounding. Recall that pet owners had a better than sixfold greater likelihood of survival in the first year following discharge from a coronary care unit than patients who were without animal companions. The authors report that their findings are consistent with the hypothesis that social affiliation and companionship have important, positive health benefits. Are there other equally plausible explanations? Are there other attributes pet owners possess that might contribute to a more favorable outlook for survival after heart attack? Several possibilities come to mind. Perhaps people who tolerate pets possess more easygoing personalities and less coronary-prone, aggressive behavior of the sort that predisposes to future cardiac problems. Or perhaps, because pets require attention and care, pet owners tend to be younger and more active than nonowners and thus more likely to survive.

Confounding factors are always in the shadows, ready to cast doubt on the interpretation of studies. The apparent link between the ingestion of lead paint and low IQ may be confounded by poor social

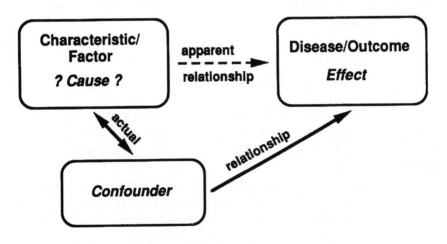

FIGURE 12-1 The confounding triangle.

environment, which is related both to intellectual underachievement and accessibility to lead paint. The improved perinatal outcomes of women utilizing the alternative birthing center may not be due to the innovative facility but to the improved outcomes to be expected from the healthier, better educated, more highly motivated volunteers who select the birthing-center option. With confounding a ubiquitous danger, savvy authors will make some effort to deal with these potential alternative explanations.

DEALING WITH CONFOUNDING

Confounding may be attacked either in the design of the study or during analysis. Matching is a technique used in the design stage. Matching, as discussed in Chap. 3, is generally utilized in observational studies. Comparison subjects are selected who share specific similarities (age, weight, race, sex) with the cases. Matched characteristics are eliminated as competing explanations of the disease. Matching before the fact is not always practical. Investigators may not be able to choose ideal controls or may not anticipate potential confounding factors in advance. Techniques are available for controlling the effects of confounding during the analysis of data. Two methods that readers will commonly encounter are control tables and multivariate analysis.

Control tables

The control-table method is stratification ex post facto. Rather than arranging subjects by age groups, smoking habits, or blood pressure levels as the study design is being created, results are calculated within specified subdivisions.

An example of a confounding relationship that has perplexed researchers is the possible link between sugar consumption and heart disease. Back in the early 1960s, Yudkin and Roddy postulated that increased intake of sucrose might lead to coronary artery disease.[2] In a case-control study, they compared 20 subjects recovering from acute myocardial infarctions with 25 controls who were either healthy or were patients on an orthopedic ward. Mean sugar intake for the two groups differed considerably, as shown in Table 12-3. Heart disease patients reported consuming almost twice as much sugar as controls. These were provocative findings and stimulated other researchers to test the hypothesis.[3-5] In the course of this subsequent work, it became apparent that individuals who consumed large amounts of sugar had other habits that might be related to heart disease. They consumed substantial amounts of coffee and tea, and they smoked more. While the issue is still not resolved to everyone's satisfaction, the relationship of smoking, which most researchers agree is a risk factor for heart disease, to sugar consumption has created a confounding problem. For purposes of illustration, let us use some hypothetical data to see how this confounding might work.

Yudkin's figures show that heart disease patients consume an average of 132 g of sugar per day, compared with 77 g daily for controls. If, however, people who eat more sugar also smoke more, and smokers are apportioned differently among cases and controls, the results might appear as in Table 12-4. The overall averages reflect the apparent association; but by evaluating sugar intake within subgroups of smoking and nonsmoking subjects, the effects of smoking are controlled. Once this is done, the relationship between sugar consumption and heart disease disappears. Mean sugar consumption for heart disease patients who smoke is almost identical to that of smoking control patients. Likewise, nonsmokers consume only 50 g of sucrose per day regardless of whether or not they have heart disease. Smoking is related to heart disease; sucrose intake is not. It is apparent, however, that for the relationship between sucrose

---

• **TABLE 12-3** •

Mean daily sugar consumption of 20 patients with heart disease and 25 control subjects

	Sugar consumption, g /day
Heart disease patients ($n = 20$)	132
Control subjects ($n = 25$)	77

SOURCE: Based on data from Yudkin and Roddy.[2]

· TABLE 12-4 ·	
Mean daily sugar consumption of 20 patients with heart disease and 25 control subjects	
	Sugar consumption, g/day
Heart disease patients ($n = 20$)	132
Smokers ($n = 16$)	152
Nonsmokers ($n = 4$)	50
Control subjects ($n = 25$)	77
Smokers ($n = 7$)	148
Nonsmokers ($n = 18$)	50

and heart disease to completely disappear, smokers must be very unevenly distributed. Of the 20 heart attack patients, 16 must be smokers, compared with only 7 of the 25 controls, to achieve the results that were obtained.

Frequently, a confounding factor exerts an influence on results but is not entirely responsible for findings. When Elwood et al. attempted to replicate Yudkin's work, they found that smoking indeed confounded the relationship between sugar consumption and heart disease, but that even when smoking was controlled, a small residual relationship remained.[5] Table 12-5 depicts two different ways our hypothetical data can be displayed. Both formats are encountered in medical articles and are referred to as *control tables*. Table 12-5(b) looks just like the two-by-two tables we used before to categorize subjects by diseases and characteristics, but it is a bit more complex. It shows the relationship between three rather than two variables. The figures in each box no longer represent the number of subjects, they portray an attribute of the subjects—in this case, mean daily sugar consumption. Reading the rows of the control table, comparing smokers with nonsmokers, we find that regardless of whether subjects have heart disease or not, smokers have higher sugar consumption (152 g/day compared with 101 g/day, 118 g/day compared with 50 g/day). Inspecting the columns, we see that patients with heart disease also consume more sugar than patients without heart disease in both the smoking and the nonsmoking groups. The conclusion to be drawn from this table is that the relationship between sugar consumption and

• TABLE 12-5 •
Mean daily sugar consumption for 20 patients with heart disease and 25 control subjects (controlled for smoking)

	Sugar consumption, g/day
(a)	
Heart disease patients ($n = 20$)	132
Smokers ($n = 12$)	152
Nonsmokers ($n = 8$)	101
Control subjects ($n = 25$)	77
Smokers ($n = 10$)	118
Nonsmokers ($n = 15$)	50

(b)

	Sugar consumption, g/day	
	Heart disease	Controls
Smokers	152 ($n = 12$)	118 ($n = 10$)
Nonsmokers	101 ($n = 8$)	50 ($n = 15$)

heart disease is in fact confounded by smoking. But when the effect of smoking is held constant, the association between sucrose consumption and heart disease remains. Both smoking and sugar are related to heart problems.

Multivariate analysis

Control tables are dandy for handling confounding variables when only one or two of the confusing factors are around. However, in many situations, a number of explanations are competing for causation credit. Human behavior is complex business. Heart disease has been linked to age, diet, personality type, blood pressure, cigarette smoking, and cholesterol level. Pregnancy outcome has been shown to be related to maternal age, race, socioeconomic status, parity, and marital status, to mention a few. Many of these causal factors are interrelated. When it comes time to sort out just what is responsible for an outcome or effect, simple control tables are not up to the task. By the time we have tried to compare the sugar consumption of subjects who are of the same sex and age, smoke the same amount, have similar cholesterol levels, and have the same range of blood pressure, life has become exceedingly complex. The more factors we control in a data analysis, the smaller the number of subjects becomes in each subdivision and the larger samples must be to avoid incorrect inferences.

The multivariate regression models discussed in Chap. 9 are useful in this situation. When the relationship between survival after discharge from the coronary care unit and pet ownership was being explored, the authors realized that a number of factors govern prognosis following heart attack.[1] Among the most important of these are the subject's age and the complications surrounding the cardiac event. In an attempt to decide just where pets fit into this complex prognostic scheme, the investigators employed a discriminant function analysis to control for physiological severity, age, mood, support, and social isolation. They did so to corral variables that might be related both to heart disease and pet ownership. Although it turns out that having a pet is not nearly so potent a predictor of survival as the physiological severity of the initial heart attack, pets made a contribution to outcome that was independent of the other factors considered.

Remember, the fact that the discriminant function analysis showed that pet ownership played a statistically significant role in survival does not necessarily mean that discharge orders for cardiac patients should include advice to purchase a dog or cat. Results of this particular study indicate that only 2.5 percent of the total variance is explained by pet ownership. This means that in the multivariate mathematical model used to predict survival, pet ownership has only a small predictive role.

One last point. Simply using sophisticated multivariate techniques to sort out multiple possible explanations of a phenomenon does not guarantee success. The authors of the pet study postulate that pet ownership is directly linked to survival by the protective effects of companionship. We need not be convinced. Pet ownership may still be a proxy for some unidentified attributes shared by people who will have more favorable outcomes following heart attack. The authors may not have thought to include them in the statistical model.

MAKING ASSOCIATIONS
INTO CAUSES

Tracking causes more often takes us through a labyrinth of tangled streets than down a straight path. When we have stripped away bias, chance, and confounders and convinced ourselves that an exposure factor or intervention is directly and independently linked to a disease or outcome, we still may not have a complete picture. Even if we are convinced that Reye syndrome is directly related to aspirin ingestion, what is the exact cause of the illness? Does the drug act as a direct liver toxin? Why do only a handful of children who take aspirin contract the disease? Is the illness a response to a mix of factors including host susceptibility, concurrent viral illness, and the drug? The causes of even seemingly straightforward infectious diseases are surprisingly complex. It is overly simple, for example, to say that tuberculosis is caused by the tubercle bacillus. While the infecting organism must be present for tuberculosis to occur, only 10 to 15 percent of individuals who are infected with the germ ever develop active tuberculosis. The bacillus is a necessary but not a sufficient cause for the illness. Host resistance, nutritional status, social isolation, and adaptability to stress also play a role. Discussions of cause can rapidly become metaphysical as well as biological. For readers who are interested in detailed discussions of the subject, some thought-provoking reviews are available.[6,7]

For practical purposes, most clinicians have a threshold at which the evidence for etiology is strong enough to elicit action. John Snow reportedly dismantled the Broad Street pump to curtail the cholera that was raging in mid-nineteenth-century London when he became convinced of the causal role that water played in the epidemic; but his action preceded the identification of the cholera vibrio, which most would consider the cause of cholera, by several decades.

There are several practical hints that clinician readers can use to help decide whether the associations they read about are causal enough to precipitate action. Hill has published a classic essay on causation.[8] He speaks of nine features of relationships that are useful in constructing a case for causation. These are summarized in Table 12-6. At the risk of repetition, it is worth elaborating on some of these points in more detail.

• **TABLE 12-6** •

Features of associations that support causation

1. Strength of the association
2. Consistency of the observed evidence
3. Specificity of the relationship
4. Temporality of the relationship
5. Biological gradient of the dose-response
6. Biological plausibility
7. Coherence of the evidence
8. Experimental confirmation
9. Reasoning by analogy

SOURCE: Based on Hill.[8]

Strength of the association

One bit of evidence that tips the association balance toward causality is the strength of the association. When the relative risk or relative odds are high, the argument for cause gains support. The over-employed but potent example used to illustrate the point is the association between cigarette smoking and lung cancer. Here, odds ratios as high as 30 to 1 have been found. The statement that a heavy cigarette user is 30 times more likely to contract lung cancer than a nonsmoker is difficult to ignore. On the other hand, the case for causation is weakened when the magnitude of risk is low.

Dose-response relationship

Anytime a risk factor comes in doses or gradients of exposure, it is reasonable to expect that the risk of disease should increase with higher levels of exposure. Again, cigarette smoking and lung cancer provide the perfect example, as the work of Doll and Hill[9] shows (see Fig. 12-2). The more cigarettes people smoke, the more death rates from cancer go up and that implies causality.

This same type of evidence has been used to strengthen the ties between postmenopausal use of estrogens and development of endometrial cancer. Weiss et al. have shown that the risk of cancer is greater in women who have taken high-estrogen-content medication than for

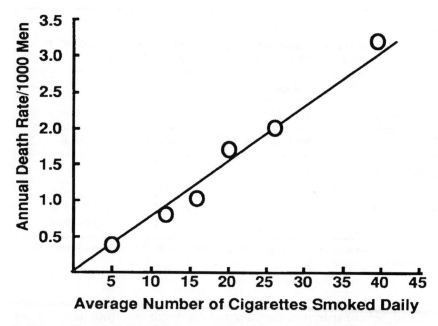

FIGURE 12-2 Annual death rate per 1000 men by average number of cigarettes smoked daily. (From Doll and Hill.[9] Reprinted by permission.)

those who have consumed a lesser amount.[10] Table 12-7 demonstrates the rise in relative risk associated with increasing daily dosage. On the other hand, the lack of a biological gradient or dose-response relationship where one might expect it should give pause for thought. Several studies have attempted to establish a causal relationship between ingestion of artificial sweeteners and the development of bladder cancer.[11-13] Findings have been inconsistent. Among the pieces of puzzle that have failed to fit together are those showing increased risk of cancer as intake of artificial sweeteners increases. Table 12-8 displays the data from one case-control study comparing estimates of intake of artificial sweeteners in patients with bladder cancer and controls.[12] Although there is some indication that increasing intake of sweeteners is associated with increased risk of cancer in men, the trend is actually reversed for women.

Biological plausibility

To make a convincing argument for causation, the associations developed in medical studies should make biological sense. This means they

• TABLE 12-7 •
Menopausal estrogen use in women with endometrial cancer and controls according to average daily dosage

| Average dosage, mg/day | % of subjects | | Relative risk | 95% confidence interval |
	Endometrial cancer (*n*=309)	Control (*n*=272)		
Never used	20	63	1.0	...
≤0.5	5	7	2.5	1.1–5.3
0.6–1.2	32	12	8.8	5.0–12.7
≥1.25	44	18	7.6	5.0–11.6

SOURCE: From Weiss et al.[10] Copyright 1979, American Medical Association. Reprinted by permission.

should be consistent with information available from the related worlds of physiology, pharmacology, and anatomy. One argument that strengthens the case for estrogens as a cause for endometrial cancer has been the demonstration of concordance between the duration of exposure and development of disease. What we know of neoplasia suggests that cancers are not triggered immediately on exposure to a carcinogen but develop after a latent period. We would expect that women exposed to estrogens would contract the neoplasm only some years after initial exposure. Table 12-9 depicts the increasing relative risk associated with the length of time since women were first exposed

• TABLE 12-8 •
Relative risk of bladder cancer by level of exposure to artificial sweetners

| Relative risk | Level of exposure | | |
	Low	Medium	High
Men	1.1	1.4	1.0
Women	1.2	0.7	0.7

SOURCE: Modified from Kessler and Clark.[12]

• **TABLE 12-9** •

**Menopausal estrogen use in women with endometrial cancer
and controls according to time since first use**

Average dosage, mg/day	% of subjects		Relative risk	95% confidence interval
	Endometrial cancer (n = 281)	Control (n = 251)		
Never used	22	68	1.0	...
1–2	2	4	1.2	0.4–3.7
3–4	7	4	5.4	2.5–11.5
5–7	14	9	4.7	2.6–8.4
8–10	19	6	11.7	6.2–21.8
11–14	20	3	24.2	11.8–49.4
15–19	13	4	10.2	5.3–20.0
≥20	4	1	8.3	2.8–24.5

SOURCE: From Weiss et al.[10] Copyright 1979, American Medical Association. Reprinted by permission.

to estrogens. Women with less than 3 years on the medication have essentially no increased risk of cancer.

Results are sometimes called into question because of apparent gaps in biological plausibility. Interpretations of data from the anturane reinfarction trial have been complicated by findings that seem inconsistent with the properties of the drug under study.[14] The purpose of this large controlled trial was to see if sulfinpyrazone, a drug that inhibits platelet aggregation, would prove useful in preventing death among patients recovering from heart attack. This multicenter study compared mortality rates of over 1500 patients who had suffered myocardial infarction and were randomized to receive either sulfinpyrazone or placebo. After 24 months of follow-up, the sulfinpyrazone group had experienced approximately 32 percent less cardiac mortality than placebo-treated patients, a finding that "borders on conventional levels of statistical significance ($p = 0.058$)."

However, close inspection of the results revealed that this difference was due almost entirely to prevention of sudden death (presumably due to arrhythmias) rather than of recurrent myocardial infarction. In fact, reinfarction rates for the two groups were identical. This was an unexpected finding, and it does not fit with the postulated beneficial effect of sulfinpyrazone. The drug is supposed to prevent platelet aggregation and subsequent reinfarction, not prevent arrhythmias. So while the medication appears to work, it works for the wrong reasons. Perhaps further research will demonstrate a perfectly plausible explanation for these seemingly implausible results. In the meantime, one cannot help but withhold unbridled enthusiasm for sulfinpyrazone until the mechanism by which it obtains its protective effects is clarified.

Consistency of the observed evidence

Evidence ought to hang together in a consistent manner, both within the confines of a study and from one study to another. An additional mark against the possible causal relationship between artificial sweeteners and bladder cancer is made by the inconsistency of the data. While weak associations have been noted between sweeteners and cancer in some of the case-control studies undertaken,[11,13] significant findings have been limited to subgroups of the population. In one early study, investigators found an increased risk of 1.6 for bladder neoplasms in men who ingested sugar substitutes.[11] However, this relationship was not seen for women, who had a risk of less than 1 (0.6). In a more recent article,[13] the results were reversed. The slight excess risk that could be attributed to artificial sweeteners was demonstrated only for women and not for men (relative risks of 1.6 and 0.8, respectively). This inconsistency, together with the low strength of association that was found, weakens the case for cause.

If an association between a factor and a disease is demonstrated time and time again through a number of studies that utilize different populations and different study techniques, the argument for causation is improved. Once more the smoking/lung cancer story serves as a paradigm. The evidence for causation just keeps growing. The association is demonstrated in case-control studies in which patients with lung cancer admit to substantially higher use of cigarettes than controls. It is also seen in follow-up studies, such as those of British doctors conducted by Doll and Hill.[9]

SUMMARY

The search for causation is always under the ominous shadow of confounding factors. Characteristics that seem directly related to outcomes or diseases may be incorrectly identified as causal because of linkages with intermediary, confounding variables. Careful readers should ask:

1. Have the authors addressed the possibility that chance, bias, or confounding factors are responsible for the effects they have observed?

2. Have steps been taken to control confounding? Was matching employed when the study design was created, or have multivariate techniques or control tables been employed in the analysis?

3. If authors have supplied evidence that potentially causal factors are not confounded, what additional evidence is there to suggest causality? Does evidence of the strength of the association, the biological plausibility, the consistency, and the dose-response relationship make a convincing case?

REFERENCES

1. Friedmann E, Katcher AH, Lynch JJ, Thomas SA: Animal companions and one-year survival of patients after discharge from a coronary care unit. *Public Health Rep* 95:307, 1980.
2. Yudkin J, Roddy J: Levels of dietary sucrose in patients with occlusive atherosclerotic disease. *Lancet* 2:6, 1964.
3. Bennett AE, Doll R, Howell RW: Sugar consumption and cigarette smoking. *Lancet* 1:1011, 1970.
4. Burns-Cox, CJ, Doll R, Ball KP: Sugar intake and myocardial infarction. *Br Heart J* 31:485, 1969.
5. Elwood PC, Waters WE, Moore S, Sweetnam P: Sucrose consumption and ischemic heart disease in the community. *Lancet* 1:1014, 1970.
6. Rothman KJ: Causes. *Am J Epidemiol* 104:587, 1976.
7. Susser M: *Causal Thinking in the Health Sciences: Concepts and Strategies of Epidemiology.* New York, Oxford University Press, 1973.

8. Hill AB: *Principles of Medical Statistics*. New York, Oxford University Press, 1971.
9. Doll R, Hill AB: Mortality in relation to smoking: Ten years' observations of British doctors. *Br Med J* 1:1399, 1964.
10. Weiss NS, Szekely DR, English DR, Schweid AI: Endometrial cancer in relation to patterns of menopausal estrogen use. *JAMA* 242:261, 1979.
11. Howe GR, Burch JD, Miller AB, et al: Artificial sweeteners and human bladder cancer. *Lancet* 2:578, 1977.
12. Kessler II, Clark JP: Saccharin, cyclamate, and human bladder cancer: No evidence of an association. *JAMA* 240:349, 1978.
13. Morrison AS, Buring JE: Artificial sweeteners and cancer of the lower urinary tract. *N Engl J Med* 302:537, 1980.
14. Anturane Reinfarction Trial Research Group: Sulfinpyrazone in the prevention of sudden death after myocardial infarction. *N Engl J Med* 302:250 1980.

CHAPTER THIRTEEN

CASE SERIES, EDITORIALS, AND REVIEWS

We are constantly misled by the ease with which our minds fall into the ruts of one or two experiences.

SIR WILLIAM OSLER

$\mathcal{W}$e have devoted a good bit of energy to critical evaluation of research studies that look for explanations or that evaluate therapy. In doing so, we have neglected the large numbers of studies that we classified as descriptive back in Chap. 2. By "descriptive," we refer to papers in which authors review their experience trying to cope with diagnostically related groups, or where they catalog the depressed patients who present to their family practice clinic. The goal of these is not to explore hypotheses about cause or to test a new treatment but to share experience that may be useful to readers. The prototype of these descriptions is the case report or case series, in which groups of patients are classified and summarized according to their blood pressure, electrocardiographic changes, length of hospital stay, or any of a multitude of features of interest. We noted earlier that a case series may be the first step toward more sophisticated research.

CASE SERIES

Exceptions to the rule

Sometimes a series of cases is all that is needed to shatter a shibboleth or demonstrate exceptions to a rule. Case reports can announce the occurrence of previously unsuspected adverse drug effects or show that joggers are not immune from heart attacks. Timeliness is usually a feature of this use of the case series. The information provided is often preliminary and methodologically unrefined, but it has a legitimate place in journal pages because it is "newsworthy."

In the midst of great public concern over the "epidemic" use of cocaine in the United States, Isner et al.[1] worried that there was a misperception that the drug is "not associated with serious medical complications." The authors describe seven cases of young adults who experienced ventricular fibrillation, myocarditis, and myocardial infarction associated with cocaine use. Their message is simple: "Recreational cocaine use may be very dangerous." The authors caution against interpreting the associations as establishing a clean, causal relationship between cocaine and cardiovascular disorders. They admit that their evidence is circumstantial. Without a denominator, we have no idea what proportion of all cocaine users these seven cases represent. Without comparisons, we cannot be certain that the number of cardiac events Isner et al. describe is not simply the expected rate in the overall population of young adults, regardless of their exposure to cocaine. Interpretation must proceed with caution. Still, the readership becomes more attentive to the possible cardiotoxicity of cocaine.

Natural history of disease

There are other ways that descriptive, case-series studies can be useful. Let us suppose that you have a 16-year-old patient who was released from the hospital only 2 weeks ago after receiving 10 days of antibiotic treatment for bacterial meningitis. He returns with a 2-day history of fever, diarrhea, and headache. Both the patient and his parents are concerned that the meningitis has returned, despite the vigorous therapy he received with the best your antibiotic arsenal had to deliver. You elect to perform a lumbar puncture and find that the fluid contains 280 white blood cells (WBCs), 76 percent of which are polymorphs. His spinal fluid glucose level is 58 mg/dL, protein level is 28 mg/dL, and Gram stain is negative. These results are puzzling. There are many fewer WBCs than on his initial lumbar puncture 3 weeks ago, but the fluid has not returned to "normal." You consult several colleagues, who offer differing opinions. One suggests that it is perfectly acceptable to see WBCs in fluid after uneventful recovery from meningitis, but another is adamant that the picture points to a recurrence of the infection. How many WBCs could one expect to see at this stage if the patient were recovering properly? What about the high percentage of polys? Has the patient's infection resolved? Has it relapsed? Or does he have a new infection? What we need is some guide to the natural history of cerebrospinal fluid (CSF) findings in appropriately treated cases of bacterial meningitis.

Fortunately your medical librarian is able to produce a paper describing a large series of cases from a well-known medical center that may be helpful. Durack and Spanos[2] reviewed 165 cases of bacterial meningitis in which results of posttreatment lumbar punctures were available. They have summarized and published their findings in a useful format. Table 13-1 shows their results. The table provides median, 95th percentile, and range data for CSF glucose, protein, leukocytes, and polymorphonuclear leukocyte percentage among patients who had lumbar punctures performed shortly after the completion of antimicrobial therapy.

• TABLE 13-1 •
Cerebrospinal fluid values of 163 patients[a] after successful treatment of bacterial meningitis

	Median	5th–95th percentiles	Range
Glucose, mg/dL	52	34–71	16–130
Protein, mg/dL	38	17–110	11–552
White blood cells/mm³	17	0–220	0–480
Percent polymorphonuclear	0	0–55	0–98

[a] Not all tests were performed in every case.

SOURCE: Modified from Durack and Spanos.[2]

Comparing the values we have obtained from our patient with those listed in the table, we find that our patient's glucose and protein levels present little cause for concern. However, the finding of 280 leukocytes, of which 76 percent are polys, is disturbing. Durack and Spanos found a median value of only 17 leukocytes in their posttreatment patients, and usually there were no polys. Our patient's values do fall within the total range these investigators observed, but, as seen in the second column, both total leukocytes and percent polys for our patient are above the reported 95th percentiles.

We must observe some caution in relating our case to these findings. Most lumbar punctures Durack and Spanos describe were done within 1 or 2 days of completing treatment, and our patient is 2 weeks posttherapy. Further, while this case series describes a broad age range of patients, from infants to adults, three-quarters of the cases were children less than 15 years old, and almost half of the cases were due to *Haemophilus influenzae*. We need to ask ourselves how much considerations of age, organism type, and length of time to repeat lumbar puncture might influence the findings. The study does not offer a breakdown of findings specific to our particular patient.

Nevertheless, this collected experience provides a more reasonable guide than the undocumented recollections of our colleagues. Although CSF glucose and protein levels are unremarkable, the WBC findings are not usual. It seems unlikely that we are dealing with the uncomplicated, natural history of recovery from bacterial meningitis.

Health services planning

Let us now shift age groups and suppose that we have been appointed to a committee to plan a new geriatrics unit for the hospital. In the course of meetings, questions arise concerning staffing needs and service requirements for the new unit. What will be the anticipated length of stay for a typical patient? What disabilities will patients have, and how frequently will these occur? Will patients need help with their daily activities? Will impaired mental status be a problem, necessitating special supervision? A study published by Warshaw et al.[3] provides guidelines to answer some of these questions. Though technically this study employs a prevalence or cross-sectional design that relates increasing age to increasing functional disability, much of its value lies in documenting the types and extent of functional impairment among hospitalized elderly. The paper reports on a survey conducted in a 400-bed community hospital. Over 250 patients aged 70 years or above were assessed on functional variables such as mental status, impaired hearing and vision, and ability to perform activities of daily living. Demographic information and features of the hospitalization such as length of stay and services required were also documented. Selected results are shown in Table 13-2.

These findings could be useful to our committee. Warshaw et al. found that the average elderly patient stayed in the hospital 21 days, with a range from 2 to 126 days. Of these patients, 34 and 40 percent had hearing and vision impairment, respectively. Many needed help with eating or dressing, including over 50 percent of the 39 patients who were 85 years of age or older. Fifty percent of patients had exhibited some degree of mental confusion, a problem that was also more prevalent among the oldest patients. We need to plan accordingly.

The personal experience of any one of us is limited, no matter how many our years of practice. Reports of series of cases enlarge our experience with only a few flips of the page. Moreover, our recollections of the details of the cases we have seen dim with time. Often they are selected by the dramatic episode rather than guided by the usual instance. We are more likely to recall the one or two cases of Stevens-Johnson syndrome that occurred after sulfonamide was given for a urinary tract infection than the 100 uneventful courses of the drug. The 165 posttreatment lumbar punctures are more than most of us are likely to collect in a career. The precise ranges and percentiles of cell counts and glucose determinations reported by Durack and Spanos provide objective data that we could never cull from our memories. We might remember the hospital experiences of some of our elderly patients, but we are unlikely to recall that the average length of stay

· TABLE 13-2 ·						
Functional impairment among 279 hospitalized elderly patients						
			Needing assistance		Impaired	
Confused	Incontinent	Confined to chair or bed	Eating	Dressing	Vision	Hearing
50%	21%	33%	38%	53%	40%	34%

SOURCE: Based on data from Warshaw et al.[3]

in this population reaches 3 weeks or that as many as 50 percent of these patients have some degree of confusion. The case series broadens our view and sharpens our faulty memories.

At the same time, we must remember important critical concerns such as external validity. Do patients from the medical center behave like those I care for? Is there any reason to believe that their cases of meningitis are any more or less severe or respond to treatment differently from those in patients I treat? Are the elderly admitted to the community hospital where Warshaw et al. worked typical of my setting? Do my patients tend to be as old, stay as long, or have the same proportion of orthopedic and urological problems? We must have some indication that these study populations are similar to our own before we can feel comfortable embracing the findings of these descriptive studies.

Therapy

We have stated that one feature of the case series is that it does not pretend to evaluate treatments. That rule is often broken. There are many reports of new operations, drug regimens, or health service improvements in which a series of patients is subjected to an intervention and our insistence on a proper control group is ignored. To be sure, there are instances in which treatment of a series of patients produces such dramatic results that even serious skeptics are won over and their cries of protest are temporarily silenced. The effects of insulin on diabetic hyperglycemia, of penicillin on pneumococcal pneumonia, or of vitamin B_{12} on pernicious anemia have been accepted without demands for randomized trials. However, these examples of "slam-bang effects," as Moses[4] calls them, are not common. Moreover, there is a grave risk that uncontrolled case-series studies will proclaim "slam-bangers" when they should not. Reports of internal mammary artery ligation for angina, gastric freezing for peptic ulcer disease, and DES for threatened abortion all broke loudly on the scene. Now each is only a whispered embarrassment of the past.

Bailar et al. include case-series studies in a discussion of "studies without internal controls."[5] They argue that studies that lack simultaneously followed comparison subjects almost always have "implicit controls." These include historic controls such as patients from the same clinic who had the older method of gallbladder surgery or community controls such as the percentage of patients in the county who had rubella in the year prior to the introduction of the new vaccine. Sometimes these "external controls" come from previously published reports on the same issue. Sometimes they are culled from "common knowledge," implying there is standard agreement, for example, that prior to the introduction of penicillin, all patients with subacute bacterial endocarditis died from the disease. We have discussed the frailties of the nonconcurrent, nonrandomized comparison subject enough so that these "implicit controls" must be viewed with skepticism. On the other hand, some useful information about new treatments can come from case-series studies.

Feasibility A case series is a reasonable way to find out whether a new intervention is feasible. Is an innovative surgical procedure technically possible? Can patients tolerate a new cancer therapeutic agent? Can home health care be provided for terminally ill patients at a reasonable cost?

When Mecklenburg et al.[6] monitored the use of insulin infusion pumps in their diabetic patients, assessing the feasibility of the technology was a principal goal. They wished to see if patients could manage insulin pumps at home over an extended period of time, whether control of glycemia could be maintained, and what problems would be encountered. The authors report their experience with 100 of their patients for up to 15 months. No comparison group treated by conventional methods of insulin administration is included. Blood sugar levels and glycosylated hemoglobin concentrations are compared before and after pump therapy is initiated.

The findings support the feasibility of using insulin pumps. Average levels of fasting and nonfasting sugar and glycosylated hemoglobin improved after patients began using the insulin pumps. These improvements were sustained over 10 months of use. Only 4 episodes of ketoacidosis and 5 episodes of serious hypoglycemia occurred. Few patients abandoned use of the pump, and there were 5 instances of pump failure. Ten patients acquired skin infections at the injection sites that required antibiotic therapy, but no permanent injuries resulted.

As far as the investigators are concerned, "the insulin infusion pump can be successfully employed in clinical practice to improve metabolic control..."[6] The technology is feasible. However, they are the first to point out that factors besides the method of insulin delivery may have influenced metabolic control. "Home glucose monitoring, intensive education, support by professional staff, and the patient's enthusiasm for a new technique were other important factors tending to enhance diabetes control."[6] The results of the study suggest the use of the insulin pump is practical, but they do not indicate whether the technology is superior to conventional insulin therapy. Other investigators have tackled this question in controlled clinical trials and found mixed results.[7-9]

Potential effectiveness Randomized clinical trials are difficult to organize and are usually costly. Some indication of effectiveness of a new intervention must be available before elaborate studies can be justified. The case series can serve this preliminary screening function.

Many anecdotes supporting the effectiveness of amygdalin (Laetrile) in the treatment of cancer spawned passionate debate among lay persons and health professionals over licensing and use of the drug.[10] Amygdalin is a natural, cyanide-containing derivative of apricot pits, and has been used as an ingredient in herbal medications for centuries. The U.S. Food and Drug Administration refused to approve the use of Laetrile despite the testimonials of many cancer patients that they had obtained remarkable beneficial effects. Because opinions about Laetrile were so divided, the National Cancer Institute sponsored a large case-series study to see if any beneficial effect of the compound could be demonstrated.

Investigators from four major medical centers across the country collaborated to assess Laetrile's potential. Patients enrolled in the study had histologically proven cancer for which no standard, effective treatment was available. They were accepted only if they were ambulatory, able to maintain oral nutrition, and in generally good condition. To be eligible, each patient had to have a tumor area that could be objectively measured. Laetrile therapy was guided by the practices described by proponents of the drug. Dosages and methods of administration were chosen to be representative of current practice, and adjuvant "metabolic therapy" diets, including high-dose vitamins and pancreatic enzymes, were added so as to parallel programs used by practitioners of Laetrile therapy. To assess results of treatment, objective criteria for response, stability, or progression of disease based on tumor size and metastatic involvement were defined. By selecting basically "healthy" cancer victims, using the full doses and adjuvant treatment recommended by Laetrile practitioners, and establishing

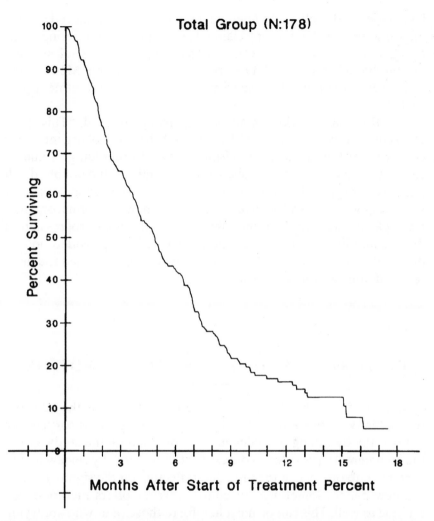

FIGURE 13-1 Patients' survival measured from the start of amygdalin treatment. (From Moertel et al.[10] Reprinted by permission of the *New England Journal of Medicine.*)

objective guidelines to measure response, investigators intended to maximize the opportunity to detect benefits of the treatment.

The results were compelling. A total of 179 patients was entered into the study. By the completion of 3 weeks of intravenous amygdalin therapy, 54 percent of the 175 evaluable patients had measurable progression of their disease. Three months after initiation of therapy, 91 percent demonstrated disease progression; by 7 months, disease had progressed in all. Only 7 percent of patients with impaired performance status prior to therapy claimed any improvement during treatment, and only 20 percent claimed any symptomatic relief anytime during therapy. Survival data were no more promising. Median survival of all patients was less than 5 months from start of treatment (Fig. 13-1).

As Relman remarked in an accompanying editorial, "This study closes the books on Laetrile."[11] The research, born out of urgent public concern that the medical establishment was "withholding" valuable cancer therapy, was not controlled, not randomized, and not blind. All patients were given Laetrile, and both patients and investigators knew what drug was being administered. In a "triumph of pragmatism over principle, it [the study] got the job done."[11] The rapid progression of disease and limited survival of the cancer patients provided no evidence of beneficial effect. The case-series results precluded the need for randomized, controlled trials.

EDITORIALS AND LETTERS TO THE EDITOR

A section of a medical journal that we have slighted is the editorial pages. Many journal editors highlight a paper they feel is particularly noteworthy by calling on colleagues to comment on the study. Often the commentary provides a context for the research by reviewing the current state of work in the area and reflecting on the significance of the new paper. Sometimes an editorial writer offers methodologic critique as well. This can be most helpful to those of us who are trying to assess the merits of a study.

Recall from Chap. 3 that *JAMA* published two articles in the same issue that took opposing points of view on the relationship between tampon use and toxic shock syndrome. Investigators from the Centers for Disease Control found the evidence compelling in favor of the relationship,[12] while the group from Yale felt that potential biases "prevent the information from being accepted as scientifically convincing."[13]

To arbitrate the dispute, a respected epidemiologist was invited to write a commentary.[14] The resulting editorial provides a detailed critique of potential methodological problems in case-control studies and assesses the likelihood that theoretical biases that threaten the validity of the studies are likely to have occurred in the toxic-shock research. After a carefully balanced discussion, she concludes, "from these perspectives, only substantial new research evidence evoking alternative explanations for existing observations would be sufficient to negate the association between TSS in menstruating women and tampon use."[14] Editorials can help readers not only to formulate opinions about the topic under debate but also to learn how to critique research from experts in the field.

Reports of a massive clinical trial that demonstrated reductions in cholesterol levels among patients taking cholestyramine prompted both editorial commentaries and a variety of interesting letters to the journal editor. The Lipids Research Clinics Coronary Primary Prevention Trial[15] followed 3086 asymptomatic middle-aged men with primary hypercholesterolemia for an average period of 7.4 years. All were placed on a moderate cholesterol-lowering diet and half received the cholesterol-lowering drug cholestyramine. The cholestyramine-treated men showed a 24 percent reduction in coronary heart disease deaths and a 19 percent reduction in nonfatal heart attacks. The study was meticulously designed and executed, a tour de force in the business of randomized controlled trials. Most readers would find the evidence convincing, as did the national news media. The authors themselves proclaimed the study left "little doubt of the benefit of cholestyramine therapy." They went on to say that:

> These results could be narrowly interpreted to apply only to the use of bile acid sequestrants in middle-aged men with cholesterol levels above 265 mg/dL (perhaps 1 to 2 million Americans). The trial's implications, however, could and should be extended to other age groups and women and, since cholesterol levels and CHD risk are continuous variables, to others with more modest elevations of cholesterol levels.[15]

Not all interpretations of the study were so sanguine. Commentaries subsequently published in the journal demonstrated the variety of viewpoints that can be the offspring of a common parent. Commentators raised a number of methodological concerns and presented alternative interpretations of the data. Some suggested that by their magnitude, the findings fell into the trap of being statistically significant but of little clinical importance.[16–19] They argued that although the researchers found a 19 percent reduction in the risk of coronary heart disease and of nonfatal myocardial infarction, the absolute difference in levels of risk between treated patients (7 percent had one of the two events), and untreated patients (8.6 percent had one event) was not impressive. They questioned the value of treating 100 patients with cholestyramine for 7 years to prevent only 1.6 coronary deaths or heart attacks. Another critic was concerned over the assumption that results of the trial could be widely generalized to other populations.[20] The study population had been restricted to middle-aged men, whose levels of cholesterol were at or above the 95th percentile of national norms. There was no evidence in the trial to suggest that women, or individuals with more moderate levels of cholesterol, would benefit from cholestyramine. Still others offered interesting alternative explanations for the findings. It was variously suggested that results were due to decreased iron stores caused by cholestyramine,[21] iatrogenic coagulopathy induced by cholestyramine,[22] and increased alcohol consumption among patients taking cholestyramine.[23] The reader need not accept these views over those of the original authors. However, critiques often raise questions that might not have occurred to us, and sometimes the arguments are convincing enough to alter our opinions.

Letters with new data

Occasionally letters to the editor include brief summaries of the letter writer's own observations of toxic shock syndrome or experience in lowering patients' cholesterol levels.

The controversy over whether coffee is a risk factor for the development of cancer of the pancreas was discussed back in Chap. 3. Shortly after the publication of the study, criticisms similar to those which we considered concerning the appropriate choice of controls were raised in several letters to the editor.[24,25] Critics argued that if hospital control patients, many of whom had gastrointestinal problems, had reduced their coffee intake because of digestive symptoms or had been advised against the beverage by their physicians, control-group coffee intake would be spuriously low. This would mean that by comparing the controls to any group with typical coffee intake, a difference would appear.

The editors of the journal offered study authors an opportunity to respond to the criticism. The investigators reformatted their data and divided control subjects into those with and without gastrointestinal-related conditions.[26] They then recalculated the odds ratios of these subgroups. Indeed, the estimated magnitude of risk was higher for patients with gastrointestinal disorders, suggesting that these individuals reported lower coffee consumption than patients with other diseases. However, a statistically significant association between coffee consumption and the risk of pancreatic cancer remained when controls with gastrointestinal disease were excluded.

Five years later, the Boston investigative group again appeared in the letters to the editor, presenting additional data on the coffee–pancreatic cancer association.[27] In a second case-control study employing similar methods, their data suggested that a modest risk was present. However, they failed to show a consistent risk among males and females or evidence of a dose-response relationship. Their conclusion was that "These results, along with other recent studies, suggest that if there is any association between coffee consumption and cancer of the pancreas, it is not as strong as our earlier data suggested."[27]

Because letters are usually limited to brief reports and preliminary observations, they rarely include detailed methodology. Nor are letters sent out for peer review, as are more substantial works of original research. Relman has issued a caveat emptor concerning data contained in letters in an editorial entitled, "How reliable are letters?"[28] "There is a risk that uncritical readers may be misled if they fail to appreciate the tentative and incomplete nature of the evidence contained in these letters."

REVIEWS

Review articles are intended to bring clinicians up to date on the state of the art of prophylactic use of antibiotics in surgery, or of diagnosis and management of arthritis. Reviews can condense a great amount of material into a few pages. They save us the trouble of pacing the dusty stacks tracking down primary sources, and hours of reading and organizing data. Most reviews focus on content. Their aim is to present a large amount of information on a subject comprehensively and efficiently. Writers of reviews are often acknowledged as experts in their fields and frequently have conducted research themselves. But it is not enough to have command of the literature on beta blockers or thyroid function. Reviews have their own set of methodological pitfalls to trap the unwary. Writers and readers of reviews must bring along their critical appraisal skills. Reviews are particularly susceptible to biases in the selection and interpretation of the papers that comprise them.

Selection

Two review articles on the management of childhood asthma appear in the same volume of a specialty journal.[29,30] Each discusses comparative benefits and side effects of oral beta-adrenergic agents and theophylline in treating childhood asthma. Opinions differ. One pair of authors[30] declares that the oral beta$_2$ agonists appear to have little to offer when compared with theophylline. In support, they summarize a single study, comparing metaproterenol with theophylline, in which the latter drug was found more effective.[31] The other reviewers disagree.[29] They state that studies comparing beta$_2$ agonists with theophylline have yielded conflicting results. Four published trials on the topic are cited.[31-34] One, which is also cited in the first review, suggests that theophylline treatment is superior; the other three report the treatments as comparable. The evidence shifts as the selection of articles changes. Without retracing the authors' steps through the *Index Medicus* and MEDLINE, can we be sure that primary sources are adequately represented in these reviews? Do these four trials represent the extent of the literature on the topic, or are four more studies with different findings lying undiscovered in the reading room stacks?

Writers of reviews should note where they looked for primary sources and what selection criteria were used to include papers in the review. Finding all the research reports on a topic is not easy. Resources such as computerized searches may include only a portion of published work. Pertinent studies may appear in journals that are not indexed or that are simply missed by indexers because key words that are used to place papers into headings differ from those that the reviewers are using in their research. Sacks et al.[35] have noted that computer searches of the literature may yield less than two-thirds of relevant papers. They suggest the use of *Current Contents*, other reviews, and experts in the field as additional resources.

Methodological critique

Neither of the review articles on asthma offers comments on the methodological quality of the papers cited. As it turns out, all four are double-blind, randomized crossover trials. But this is not always the case. Often the literature on a topic is a methodological hodgepodge, running the gamut from opinionated case reports to sophisticated controlled trials. It is not enough for a review to summarize the findings of research studies; some comment should be made on the research design and methodological quality of the work. The results of an uncontrolled series of seven patients given Bull Durham's Extract for fatigue cannot be given equal value with a carefully controlled trial comparing Bull Durham's with Lydia Pinkham's Compound.

In reviewing the effects of anabolic steroids on athletic performance, Haupt and Rovere[36] summarize the results of more than 20 published studies. The authors cover an extensive list of issues, including effects of steroids on body weight, cardiovascular performance, and strength. As part of their review, they categorize study results according to features of experimental design such as number of subjects, presence or absence of controls, and blinding. Table 13-3 illustrates this.

• TABLE 13-3 •		
Experimental design in studies of anabolic steroids		
	Studies with significant increases in strength ($n=14$)	Studies without significant increases in strength ($n=10$)
Number of subjects		
0–20	10	4
21+	4	6
Total number of subjects	239	220
Controlled	13	20
Noncontrolled	1	0
Double blind	7	9
Single blind	4	1
Not blind	3	0

SOURCE: From Haupt and Rovere.[36]

Fourteen studies demonstrated that athletes taking anabolic steroids increased their strength; 10 showed no significant improvement. The authors note the methodologic limitations of several of the studies. One uncontrolled study had only three subjects, all of whom were championship weight lifters who were, according to the original researchers, of such a level of expertise that a comparable control group was unavailable. Of the 14 studies demonstrating improved strength among athletes, the authors note that only 7 were properly blinded to avoid the possibility of placebo effect. Of the 10 studies that failed to show a strength increase, 9 employed a proper double-blind protocol. Haupt and Rovere go on to discuss the possible effect that these limitations of design, and particularly the placebo effect, may have on interpretation of results of this research. By combining their content review with methodological critique, they help the reader interpret the results of their review.

Metaanalysis/pooling

One review technique readers should know about goes by the lofty title "metaanalysis" or, more humbly, *data pooling*. Metaanalyses critically review research studies and statistically combine their data to help answer questions that are beyond the power of single papers. And "power" is just the term to describe the value of this technique. Combining data from a number of studies increases the sample size. Larger samples mean more precise estimates of rates or risks, or—in the case of clinical trials—a lesser likelihood of a type II error. Pooling of data from several small clinical trials on the same subject may reveal a clinically important difference in treatments that the individual small trials lacked the power to detect.

Philbrick and Bracikowski[37] published a review of 14 randomized controlled trials on single-dose treatment of urinary tract infections. These studies were intended to demonstrate that a single dose was as good as lengthier treatment. Generally, they were made up of small samples of patients. The equivalence of the therapies under comparison was supported by statistical testing that failed to reject the null hypothesis—a perfect opportunity for a type II error. To assess the question of whether single-dose and multidose treatments were really comparable, Philbrick and Bracikowski pooled the findings from studies in which similar treatment regimens were employed. Before they could pool data from different studies, however, the authors created some strict guidelines for inclusion of studies in the metaanalysis. The studies had to have:

1. *Uniform diagnostic criteria.* Evidence was required that patients in the various studies had the same disease, diagnosed in the same manner—in this case a culture-proven urinary tract infection.

2. *Uniform clinical severity.* Since urinary tract infections vary in severity from asymptomatic bacteriuria to pyelonephritis with sepsis, only data that met the authors' definition of "uncomplicated" urinary tract infection were used. Patients were included regardless of the outcome of tests for antibody-coated bacteria in their urine.

3. *Similar therapy.* The treatment regimens had to include the same antibiotic given at similar dosages.

4. *Uniform outcome measures.* Posttreatment urine cultures were required for inclusion.

Only 6 of the 14 studies met all criteria for pooling. Three evaluated amoxicillin and three evaluated trimethoprim-sulfamethoxazole. Each of the six studies had concluded that single-dose and multidose therapy were of equal efficacy. Individual-study and pooled results may be seen in Table 13-4. The table shows that when data were adjusted to make them comparable for pooling, interpretations changed. In three of the studies, data were modified to meet the uniform clinical severity standard. In one instance, Philbrick and Bracikowski included patients with a positive antibody-coated bacteria test, which the original authors had excluded. In another, the metaanalysts excluded patients who had antibiotic-resistant organisms. When this was done, the difference between the cure rates of single-dose and multidose treatment became statistically significant at the .05 level. After data were pooled, the number of study subjects given amoxicillin rose to over 120 subjects each in the single-dose and multidose treatments. The 15-percentage-point difference in cure rates became both clinically and statistically significant. In this instance, the more powerful pooled results are at odds with the findings of the smaller individual studies. The pooled analysis of trimethoprim-

---

· **TABLE 13-4** ·

**Single-dose compared with multidose treatment
of urinary tract infection: Adjusted,[a]
pooled results**

| | No. cured/total, % | | |
Study	Single-dose	Multidose	p Value[b]
Amoxicillin/ampicillin			
A	38/53 (72)	37/41 (90)	.023
B	39/59 (66)	61/76 (80)	.048
C	8/11 (73)	10/12 (83)	NS
Total	85/123 (69)	108/129 (84)	.005
Trimethoprim-sulfamethoxazole			
D	17/20 (85)	15/17 (88)	NS
E	30/32 (94)	15/16 (94)	NS
F	34/41 (83)	36/40 (90)	NS
Total	81/93 (87)	66/72 (90)	NS

[a]See text for explanation.
[b]For difference between cure rates by Fisher's exact test; NS= not significant.

Source: Modified from Philbrick and Bracikowski.[37] Copyright 1985, American Medical Association, with permission.

---

sulfamethoxazole studies, on the other hand, failed to detect a significant difference in the two treatments. The 3-percentage-point difference between the 87 percent cure rate for single-dose and the 90 percent cure rate for multidose is not statistically significant, nor does it appear to be clinically important. However, the authors hasten to point out that the sample size achieved through pooling is still not large and "the possibility of a type II error remains."

The technique of metaanalysis has great potential for synthesizing research results and adding precision and power to our estimates of effect. Clearly, however, great care must be taken to see that pooling is done only among studies where there is reasonable assurance that subjects and treatments are similar. Sacks et al.[35] have provided a useful "review of reviews" in which they discuss the methodology of metaanalysis.

SUMMARY

Case-series studies, editorials, and review articles are journal offerings that can add substance to our reading fare.

1. The case series can give a first glimpse of exciting new findings or demonstrate exceptions to the rule. These descriptive studies can provide data on the natural history of disease or offer experience to guide health services. The feasibility and potential effectiveness of new treatments can be evaluated. But all the interpretation risks of subject selection and absent controls attend. *Caveat emptor!*

2. Editorials and letters to the editor present thought-provoking alternative interpretations and methodological insights. They may also give testimony to the wit, good humor, and even poetic talent of our colleagues.

3. Reviews offer efficient reading, but ask yourself *(a)* Have the authors performed a thorough literature review or presented only selected research findings? *(b)* Have they accepted the primary researchers' interpretation of study data uncritically, or do they include methodological commentary along with their content review?

REFERENCES

1. Isner JM, Estes NAM III, Thompson PD, et al. Acute cardiac events temporally related to cocaine abuse. *N Engl J Med* 315:1438, 1986.
2. Durack DT, Spanos A: End-of-treatment spinal tap in bacterial meningitis: Is it worthwhile? *JAMA* 248:75, 1982.
3. Warshaw GA, Moore JT, Friedman SW, et al: Functional disability in the hospitalized elderly. *JAMA* 248:847, 1982.
4. Moses LE: The series of consecutive cases as a device for assessing outcomes of intervention. *N Engl J Med* 311:705, 1984.
5. Bailar JC III, Louis TA, Lavori PW, Polansky M: Studies without internal controls. *N Engl J Med* 311:156, 1984.
6. Mecklenburg RS, Benson JW, Becker NM, et al: Clinical use of the

insulin infusion pump in 100 patients with type I diabetes. *N Engl J Med* 307:513, 1982.

7. Coustan DR, Reece EA, Sherwin RS, et al: A randomized clinical trial of the insulin pump vs. intensive conventional therapy in diabetic pregnancies. *JAMA* 255:631, 1986.

8. Reeves ML, Seigler DE, Ryan EA, Skyler JS: Glycemic control in insulin-dependent diabetes mellitus: Comparison of outpatient intensified conventional therapy with continuous subcutaneous insulin infusion. *Am J Med* 72:673, 1982.

9. Schriffrin A, Belmonte MM: Comparison between continuous subcutaneous insulin infusion and multiple injections of insulin. *Diabetes* 31:255, 1982.

10. Moertel CG, Fleming TR, Rubin J, et al: A clinical trial of amygdalin (Laetrile) in the treatment of human cancer. *N Engl J Med* 306:201, 1982.

11. Relman AS: Closing the books on Laetrile. *N Engl J Med* 306:236, 1982.

12. Schlech WF III, Shands KN, Reingold AL, et al: Risk factors for development of toxic shock syndrome: Association with a tampon brand. *JAMA* 248:835, 1982.

13. Harvey M, Horwitz RI, Feinstein AR: Toxic shock and tampons: Evaluation of the epidemiologic evidence. *JAMA* 248:840, 1982.

14. Hulka BS: Tampons and toxic shock syndrome. *JAMA* 248:872, 1982.

15. Lipid Research Clinics Program: The Lipid Research Clinics Coronary Primary Prevention Trial results. *JAMA* 251:351, 1984.

16. Gimlett DM: Lipid Research Clinics Program (letter). *JAMA* 252:2546, 1984.

17. Norenberg DD: Lipid Research Clinics Program (letter). *JAMA* 252:2545, 1984.

18. Rahimtoola SH: Cholesterol and coronary heart disease: A perspective. *JAMA* 253:2094, 1985.

19. Renfrew RA: Lipid Research Clinics Program (letter). *JAMA* 252:2545, 1984.

20. Kronmal RA: Commentary on the published results of the Lipid Research Clinics Coronary Primary Prevention Trial. *JAMA* 253:2091, 1985.

21. Sullivan JL: Lipid Research Clinics Program (letter). *JAMA* 252:2547, 1984.

22. Conjalka MS, Reynolds TF: Lipid Research Clinics Program (letter). *JAMA* 252:2548, 1984.

23. Franks P: Lipid Research Clinics Program (letter). *JAMA* 252:2548, 1984.

24. Higgins I, Stolley P, Wynder EL: Coffee and cancer of the pancreas. *N Engl J Med* 304:1605, 1981.

25. Shedlofsky S: Coffee and cancer of the pancreas. *N Engl J Med* 304:1604, 1981.
26. MacMahon B, Yen S, Trichopoulos D, et al: Coffee and cancer of the pancreas. *N Engl J Med* 304:1604, 1981.
27. Hsieh C, MacMahon B, Yen S, et al: Coffee and pancreatic cancer (chapter 2). *N Engl J Med* 315:587, 1986.
28. Relman AS: How reliable are letters? *N Engl J Med* 308:1219, 1983.
29. Rachelefsky GS, Siegel SC: Asthma in infants and children—treatment of childhood asthma: Part II. *J Allergy Clin Immunol* 76:409, 1985.
30. Weinberger M, Hendeles L, Theophylline use: An overview. *J Allerg Clin Immunol* 76:277, 1985.
31. Dusdieker L, Green M, Smith GD, et al: Comparison of orally administered metaproterenol and theophylline in the control of chronic asthma. *J Pediatr* 101:281, 1982.
32. Nolan G, Mindorff C, Reilly PA, Levison H: Comparison of the long-term effect of fenoterol hydrobromide and theophylline syrups in preschool asthmatic children. *Ann Allerg* 49:93, 1982.
33. Rachelefsky GS, Katz RM, Mickey MR, Siegel SC: Metaproterenol and theophylline in asthmatic children. *Ann Allerg* 45:207, 1980.
34. Schuller DE, Oppenheimer PJ: A comparison of metaproterenol and theophylline for control of childhood asthma. *Clin Pediatr* 21:135, 1982.
35. Sacks HS, Berrier J, Reitman D, et al: Meta-analyses of randomized controlled trials. *N Engl J Med* 316:450, 1987.
36. Haupt HA, Rovere GD: Anabolic steroids: A review of the literature. *Am J Sports Med* 12:469, 1984.
37. Philbrick JT, Bracikowski JP: Single-dose antibiotic treatment for uncomplicated urinary tract infections: Less for less? *Arch Intern Med* 145:1672, 1985.

CHAPTER FOURTEEN

A FINAL WORD

"When I use a word," Humpty Dumpty said in a rather scornful tone, "it means just what I choose it to mean—neither more nor less."
"The question is," said Alice, "whether you can make words mean so many different things."
"The question is," said Humpty Dumpty, "which is to be master—that's all."

—LEWIS CARROLL, Through the Looking Glass

$\mathcal{A}$s promised, we have worked our way through the major structure of a medical article. We have sampled study designs and their strengths and weaknesses, looked at the way data are collected and at some biases that creep into that activity, and devoted considerable energy to critically evaluating the way results are presented and analyzed. Along the way we discovered many pitfalls that plague medical studies and journal articles. We uncovered biases that occur because of selective recall, loss to follow-up, and poor sampling techniques. We saw the untoward effects of observer bias, the havoc wreaked by confounding factors, and the confusion created by misinterpretation of normal distributions and statistical significance.

We have honed our critical cutlery by learning something of random allocation, stratification, control tables, and confidence intervals. In this last chapter the accent will be on mobilizing the concepts of the previous pages into a final assessment of the value of an article. After all is said and done, is the information contained within the glossy pages worth retaining? Is it information that will change practice habits or improve patient care? Is the message the authors are conveying worth our continued consideration?

It has been mentioned before but is worth repeating that medical studies are rarely free from blemish. With our sharpened critical awareness, it is possible to find a tender spot in almost any article. The trick is to put skills to work in a constructive manner, balance the good points and the flaws, and decide upon a report's overall merit. Skills in critical analysis are easily abused. Without temperance, skepticism can degenerate into nihilism. That nets very little. On the other hand, as we pass from a thorough review of a study's methodology, through a careful evaluation of the collection of data and presentation of results, to the authors' discussion, we need to have confidence in our own abilities as critical reviewers. As authors put forth their interpretation and discuss the meaning of their work, we have every right to exercise our hard-earned judgment. If cynicism is a danger, so is self-effacement. Too often readers are willing to accept the views of medical writers and editors over their own reactions. Under intimidation by the experts, common sense is put aside. That is a mistake. The question, as Humpty Dumpty puts it to Alice, is "which is to be master?"

CLARITY

Most of us have had the unsettling experience of reading an article once and then a second time only to be left with the unhappy realization that we had no idea what the author was trying to say. Most often we take this to heart as a personal shortcoming: we feel that a defect in our education or basic intellect is to blame for our failure to grasp the message. Rarely do we consider that it may be the writer's rather than the reader's deficiency. Medical articles are not always clearly written. Crichton has assailed medical writers for obfuscation, for camouflaging their communication in awkward prose and unnecessary complexity.[1] He says the effect of this bad writing is to

> make medical prose as dense, impressive and forbidding as possible...the stance of authors seems designed to astound and mystify the reader with a dazzling display of knowledge and scientific acumen...what they (authors) are communicating is their profound *scientific-ness*, not whatever the title of their paper may be.[1]

Crichton's accusations that medical writers deliberately write obscurely to conceal thin papers and appear scientifically profound may smack of hyperbole, but there are seeds of truth. There is even some objective evidence to support Crichton's claims that medical minds can mistake bombast for wisdom. Researchers interested in the evaluations of medical students conducted several experiments assessing what has become known as the Doctor Fox effect.[2] In these studies, an actor was trained to lecture to medical students in a manner that would seduce them into feeling "satisfied that they had learned despite the presentation of irrelevant, conflicting, and meaningless content." The actor, dubbed "Dr. Fox," delivered his lectures with style, humor, and verve. They were, however, filled with "double talk, neologisms, non sequiturs, and contradictory statements." Students rating Dr. Fox gave his lectures highest marks in both style and content.

Impressed by the effects of the Dr. Fox experiment, Armstrong applied the principle to professional journals.[3] To test the hypothesis that "researchers who want to impress their colleagues...write less intelligible papers," he asked 20 business school faculty members to rate 10 management journals according to journal prestige. The readability of each journal was then assessed by applying a test of reading ease to sample articles. The test determined readability by sentence length and the number of syllables for each 100 words. Sure enough, there was a positive correlation between wordy, polysyllabic sentences and the estimated prestige. Because it might be argued that the content of the high-toned journals is more sophisticated and thus requires more elaborate prose, Armstrong added a second part to his experiment. He took concluding paragraphs from several articles and rewrote them, altering the readability but not the content. He sent these to another group of faculty members, asking them to rate the competence of the articles on the basis of the samples provided. Again, pedantry triumphed. Obscure writing tended to be rated higher in competence than simple, straightforward prose.

Although it may be unfair to generalize from management journals to medical writing, there is a message in this for medical readers. Clarity is the author's responsibility. If convoluted sentences and hazy verbiage obscure meaning, it is the writer's fault. Readers need to shake off the notion that their intellectual inadequacies are to blame when they have difficulty understanding a study. By the time most of us reach the stage where medical articles are appropriate reading, we are clever enough to understand them.

APOLOGIES, TENTATIVE CONCLUSIONS, SELF-CRITICISM, AND THE LIKE

It is interesting to see how authors critique their own work in the discussion and conclusion sections of articles. Some authors are supremely certain of their results, others are overly modest. Blustering self-confidence invites close scrutiny when the author "doth protest too much." Results that are truly "obvious" or "self-evident" usually do not need the additional fanfare. Investigators' self-criticisms can range from empty apologies to insightful commentaries on the merits of the work. Some discussions contain so many modifying adjectives and qualifying phrases, the study swoons from dizzy indecision. "There may seem," "it might hopefully appear," "although evidence may be lacking," and "it may be generally considered to be" head a long list of qualifiers that weaken not only the writing style but the force of the message as well. Another kind of troublesome hedging occurs when, after laboring through the entire paper, we are told that the "results are only preliminary at this time," or that "the numbers studied may be too small to extract meaningful conclusions." Qualifications like these are defended on the grounds that authors are trying not to overstate their case or make unsubstantiated claims. The intent is honest enough. Unfortunately, disclaimers that are tacked on to the final paragraphs of a piece offer readers no constructive alternatives for interpreting results. When authors quaver in their resolve, it shakes our confidence as well. We are left uncertain about the importance of the message. Do they really believe in their work? Is it useful news for clinicians? How could it be improved or made meaningful?

On the other hand, genuine constructive criticism fosters confidence. It is reassuring when authors critically analyze their methods and interpretations. In a study reporting the "decreased risk of fractures of the hip and lower forearm with post-menopausal use of estrogens," Weiss et al. head their discussion with a section entitled, "Limitations of the Data."[4] They greet potential problems in this study head-on, describing possible biases and shortcomings in their work and assessing the effects of these upon interpretation.

In collecting information from cases and controls about estrogen use, systematic differences occurred. Women who had sustained fractures (cases) were interviewed on average 1 year after the fracture had occurred. However, they were asked to report estrogen use only until the time they sustained the broken bone. Controls, on the other hand, reported estrogen use until the time of interview. The authors worried that cases might have reported less estrogen usage because of the lapses of memory that occur with time rather than because of real differences in taking the medication. To attack this problem, they reanalyzed their data after removing the potential information bias. They dropped information about control subjects' use of estrogens for the year immediately prior to interview. Lower estrogen use among women with fractures was still demonstrated, supporting the beneficial effects of estrogens.

When we see references to "potential bias in our method" or accounts of "methods for controlling potential confounders," we can tell that authors share some of our critical concerns. Most authors are vested in their research hypothesis. They believe that estrogens reduce fractures and that treating high blood pressure reduces the risk of stroke. It is encouraging when they try alternate methods of analysis and still support their hypothesis.

THE FINAL WORD

Regardless of how adamantly authors defend, support, deny, decry, declaim, apologize, or equivocate, we have a perfect right to disagree with their interpretation and offer our own. This disagreement over interpretation need not flow from problems with the paper's methods or analysis. It may simply be a matter of differing opinions over the importance of the findings reported.

Consider a large randomized study conducted in the Netherlands that assessed the value of intramuscular lidocaine for preventing fatal arrhythmias after heart attack.[5] In this elegant experiment, paramedics used automatic injectors to administer lidocaine or placebo to over 7000 patients with acute chest pain prior to transporting them to the hospital. Patients were carefully monitored for arrhythmias, with the end point being the occurrence of ventricular fibrillation within 60 min following the injection.

The authors found that only half as many patients given lidocaine experienced ventricular fibrillation compared with controls. When the comparison included only patients with fibrillation occurring 15 min or more after the injection (when therapeutic plasma levels of lidocaine had been reached), there were only 2 cases in the treated group, compared with 12 among control patients. This becomes a statistically significant and perhaps clinically important difference. However, approximately 3000 patients were enrolled in each of the study groups. In about one-third of these, a final diagnosis of myocardial infarction was made. The total number of fibrillation events was less than one-half of 1 percent of all patients transported and only 1.3 percent of patients subsequently diagnosed as having had a heart attack. Five cases of ventricular fibrillation were prevented for every 1000 heart attack patients transported. Some may find that a small rate of return.

Several of the writers who commented on the results of the Lipids Research Clinics Coronary Primary Prevention Trial disagreed with the importance of the findings in this large study.[6-8] Criticisms were based not on perceived flaws in the study design nor on the statistical analysis. Commentators differed over practical aspects of the study. We have already mentioned the criticism that cholestyramine prevented only 1.5 coronary deaths or heart attacks for every 100 patients treated. The drug is also costly and difficult to take.[7,8] Patients were required to take six 4-g packets of cholestyramine resin each day at a cost that several writers estimated between $120 and $150 per month. This means that during the 7-year course of the study, over $700,000 in drug costs will be incurred for every cardiac event prevented. Whether one feels such an expense is justified is an individual matter. But every reader must decide for any given study whether the risk averted or treatment benefit reported is valuable in the larger socioeconomic context. Authors who provide estimates of costs expended for benefits received help the reader in making this assessment. Our opinions in these matters are as important at those of the "experts."

SUMMARY

We are back where we began—with a desktop full of journals, a desire to be knowledgeable, and a distressingly tiny aliquot of time. We have learned some analytic techniques and mastered our fears of inadequacy when confronting the experts. The task is formidable but not impossible. With a little planning, perseverance, and practice, we can make the medical literature not only palatable but downright digestible.

REFERENCES

1. Crichton M: Medical obfuscation: Structure and function. *N Engl J Med* 293:1257, 1975.
2. Ware JE, Williams RG: The Dr. Fox effect: A study of lecturer effectiveness and ratings of instruction. *J Med Educ* 50:149, 1975.
3. Armstrong JS: Unintelligible management research and academic prestige. *Interfaces* 10:80, 1980.
4. Weiss NS, Ure CL, Ballard JH, et al: Decreased risk of fractures of the hip and lower forearm with postmenopausal use of estrogen. *N Engl J Med* 303:1195, 1980.
5. Koster RW, Dunning AJ: Intramuscular lidocaine for prevention of lethal arrhythmias in the prehospitalization phase of acute myocardial infarction. *N Engl J Med* 313:1105, 1985.
6. Gimlett DM: Lipid Research Clinics Program (letter). *JAMA* 252:2546, 1984.
7. Norenberg DD: Lipid Research Clinics Program (letter). *JAMA* 252:2545, 1984.
8. Renfrew RA: Lipid Research Clinics Program (*letter*). *JAMA* 252:2545, 1984.

INDEX

Abnormal, definition of, 137–39
Abstracts, 6–7
Abuse of children, surveillance bias
   and, 73–74
Age, matching technique and, 44
AIDS. *See* HIV infection.
Alcohol consumption:
   blood pressure and, 30, 150
   education of servers and, 106–7
   maternal, febrile seizures in infant
     and, 37, 43
Allocation of subjects, 99–104
Alopecia, cigar smoking and, 44,
   215–16
Alpha error, 154, 155
Alternation of subjects, 88–89
Amoxicillin:
   diarrhea and, 147
   urinary tract infections and, 80–81,
     85–86, 153–54
   pooled analysis of, 247–48
Ampicillin, diarrhea and, 147–48
Amygdalin therapy of cancer, 238–40
Anabolic steroids, athletic
   performance and, 245–46
Analysis by intention to treat, 105
Angiography, spectrum problem and,
   194
Animals:
   companion, heart disease and, 204,
     217, 222
   multiple sclerosis and, 206–9

Antecedent-consequent relationships,
   65–66
Antibiotics, single-dose, urinary tract
   infections and, 80–81, 85–86, 153–54,
   157, 246–48
Anticipation, bias and, 116–18
Anticoagulants, myocardial infarction
   and, 97, 101–2
Antihistamines, otitis media and,
   150–51
Antihypertensive agents, compliance
   in use of, 96
Anturane reinfarction trial, 227
Approaches to article, 9–12
Arrhythmias, lidocaine and, 257
Articles, 1–12
   abstract of, 6–7
   approaches to, 9–12
   clarity in, 253–55
   design of. *See* Design of study.
   discussion/conclusions sections of, 7,
     8, 255–56
   interpretation of. *See* Interpretation.
   introduction of, 7–8
   methods section of, 8, 11–12, 245–46
   reasons for reading, 4–6
   references/bibliography in, 8–9
   results section of, 8
   review, 243–48
     content, 243
     metaanalysis (data pooling) in,
       245–46

Articles, review (*cont.*):
  methodological critique in, 245–46
  selection process used by, 244
  scanning of, 10–11
  selectivity in reading of, 9–10
  structure of, 6–9
  subheadings in, 11
  summary of, 6–7
  validity of, 3–4
Artificial sweeteners, bladder cancer
  and, 225, 226, 228
Aspirin:
  myocardial infarction prevention
    and, 82, 106
  Reye's syndrome and, 39, 41–42
Assignment of subjects, 99–104
Association, 169, 223–28
  biological plausibility of, 225–28
  consistency of evidence of, 228
  diagnostic technique and, 179–84
  dose-response, 224–25
  regression analysis and, 173
  strength of, 224
Attrition:
  experimental study, 104–6
  in follow-up, 70–73
Automobile accidents:
  car seats for infants and, 119–20
  rear-seat safety and, 158
Average, 130

Bacteremia, cultures in children and,
  61–63, 179–84
Bacteriuria in schoolgirls, 28, 131–32
Baldness, cigar smoking and, 44,
  215–16
Before-and-after study, 91. *See also*
  Experimental studies.
Bell-shaped curve, 128, 129
Beta blockers, myocardial infarction
  and, 104–5
Beta errors, 154–56, 166
Bias, 50–51, 215
  allocation, 99–102
  attrition, 71, 72
  in case-control study. *See*
    Case-control studies, bias in.

cointervention, 97
compliance, 94–97
control choice and, 39–40
diagnosis, 38
double-blind trial and, 122
experimental study, 94–97
hospital as source of subjects and,
  39–40
information, 48
interviewer, 48, 118
measurement, 116–22
  familiarity and, 121–22
  investigator, 117–18
  subject, 118–22
participation, 63–65
"potential," 256
pretesting and, 122
recall, 45–47
reporting, 38
research, 47–48
response, 47, 50, 63–65
sampling, 61, 62
  in case-control study, 37, 38
selection:
  allocation and, 99, 101, 102
  spectrum problem and, 194
social desirability, 119–20
standards and, 195
statistical significance and, 158–59
subject, 45–47, 118–22
surveillance, 73–74
Bibliography, 8–9
Biological plausibility, 225–28
Biostatistics, 145. *See also* Statistical
  significance; Statistical tests.
Birth, Leboyer, 101, 104, 122
Bladder cancer, artificial sweeteners
  and, 225, 226, 228
Blood pressure. *See also* Hypertension.
  alcohol consumption and, 30, 150
  reliability of measurement of, 112
  variation in, 140–42
  weight and, 170, 173, 175
  loss of, 158
Breast cancer:
  estrogen therapy and, 47
  screening for, 195

Cancer:
  bladder, artificial sweeteners and, 225, 226, 228
  breast:
    estrogen therapy and, 47
    screening for, 195
  colorectal, CEA and, 193–94
  endometrial. *See* Endometrial cancer.
  gastric, *Helicobacter pylori* and, 48–50
  Laetrile (amygdalin) therapy of, 238–40
  lung. *See* Lung cancer.
  pancreatic, coffee consumption and, 38–40, 242–43
Carcinoembryonic antigen, colorectal cancer and, 193–94
Carotid artery surgery, TIAs or stroke and, 105–6
Case(s). *See also* Subjects.
  definition of, 28, 38–39
  matching of controls with, 43–45. *See also* Matching.
  recall bias and, 45–47
  selection of, in case-control study, 36–39
Case-control studies, 20–21, 34–52
  advantages of, 35–36
  bias in, 50–51
    control choice and, 39–40
    information, 48
    recall, 45–47
    research, 47–48
    sampling, 37, 38
    subject, 45–47
  community controls and, 42–43
  data bases and, 36
  definition of case in, 38–39
  efficiency of, 35
  example of, 23–24
  exposure data in, 45–50
  frequency of use of, 34–35
  matching technique and, 43–45
    excessive application of, 45
    risk and, relative, 207–8
  misuse of term for, 28

  multiple controls in, 41–42
  nested, 48–50
  outline of, 20
  problems of, 36–51
  rare diseases and, 35
  retrospective nature of, 29
  risk and, relative, 204–9
  sampling in, 36–38
  selection of cases in, 36–39
  selection of controls in, 39–40
  time-order relationships and, 65–66
Case reports, 17
Case series, 231–39
  controls in, 236–37
  effectiveness of intervention and, 237–38
  exceptions to the rule and, 232
  feasibility and, 237–38
  health services planning and, 234–36
  natural history of disease and, 232–34
  personal experience vs., 235–36
  therapy and, 236–39
  validity of, external, 236
Categorical data, 164–66
Causes, 214–29
  biological plausibility of, 225–28
  confounding and, 215–18
    dealing with, 218–22
  consistency of evidence and, 228
  control tables and, 218–21
  dose-response relationship and, 224–25
  multivariate analysis and, 221–22
  strength of association and, 224
  summary of features supporting, 225–26
  time-order relationships and, 65–66
CEA (carcinoembryonic antigen), colorectal cancer and, 193–94
Central tendency, 130–32
Cervical dysplasia, variability in classification of, 115
Chance, 215
  chi-square test and, 164
  measurement and, 124

Chance (*cont.*):
  p value and, 149–50
  relevance of, 158
Childbirth:
  birthing-room experiment in,
    100–101
  Leboyer approach to, 101, 104, 122
Chi-square test, 164–65
  nominal data and, 165–66
Cholesterol:
  cholestyramine and, 241–42, 257
  multiple risk factor intervention
    and, 98
Cholestyramine, cholesterol levels
    and, 241–42, 257
CI (confidence interval), 156–57
Cigar smoking, baldness and, 44,
    215–16
Cigarette smoking. *See* Smoking.
Clarity, 253–55
Classification, 83–85
  diagnostic technique evaluation and,
    180–81
  discriminant scores and, 189
  efficiency of, 183
  regression to the mean and, 140–42
  sensitivity vs. specificity choice in,
    187–88
  technical procedures and, 85–87
Clinical series, 17
Clinical trials, 18, 32. *See also*
    Controlled trials; Experimental
    studies.
Clinic-based vs. population-based
    studies, 69–70
Coffee consumption:
  hospitalized vs. population-based
    groups and, 40
  pancreatic cancer and, 39–40
  letters to the editor on, 242–43
Cohort study, 22. *See also* Follow-up
    studies.
  case-control within (nested
    case-control study), 48–50
  follow-up design and, 28
  prospective nature of, 29
  retrospective, 29, 30

Cointervention, 97
Colorectal cancer, CEA and, 193–94
Comments section, 7, 8, 255–56
Community controls, 42–43, 237
Comparability among trial groups,
    90–93
Comparison subjects. *See* Controls.
Compliance, 94–97
  by controls, 97–98
Conclusions sections, 7, 8, 255–56
Concordance, 208
Confidence interval, 156–57
  continuous data and, 168
  risk and, relative, 208–9
Confidentiality, convenience sampling
    and, 63
Confounding, 215–18
  control tables and, 218–21
  dealing with, 218–22
  multivariate analysis and, 221–22
  risk ratio and, 215–16
  triangle of, 217
Continuing education, 1–2
Continuous data, 162
  confidence interval and, 168
  tests for, 166–68
Contraceptives, oral, 211–12
  postcoital, estrogen and, 90–91
Controlled trials, 18–19. *See also*
    Experimental studies.
  example of, 27
  metaanalysis (data pooling) and, 246
  outline of, 19
  prospective nature of, 29
  statistical significance vs. clinical
    importance in results of, 150–51
Controls:
  case series and, 236–37
  community, 42–43, 237
  comparability of, 90–93
  compliance by, 97–98
  crossing over vs., 88–89
  definition of, 28
  experimental, 87–93
  external, 237
  historic, 91–92, 236
  hospital as source of, 39–40, 42, 242

implicit, 236–37
internal, 236–37
mail enlistment of, 43
matching of cases with, 43–45,
    92–93. *See also* Matching.
multiple, 41–42
placebo effect and, 88–89
risk and, relative, 205
selection of, in case-control study,
    39–40
telephone enlistment of, 41, 43
Control tables, 218–21
Convenience allocation, 99–100
Convenience sample, 61, 63
Convulsions. *See* Seizures.
Cooperation, subject, 63–65
Coronary artery disease:
    cholestyramine and, 241–42, 257
    participation bias and, 64
    personality type and, 203–4
    pet ownership and, 204, 217, 222
    ventriculography and, 194
Correlation, 169–71
    coefficient of, 169, 171
        square of, 175–76
Costs, 196–98
    benefits vs., 257
Criticism, 256–57
Crossover, 88–89
Cross-sectional studies, 22–23,
    55–67
    advantages of, 58
    applications of, 58
    bias in:
        response, 63–65
        sampling, 61, 62
    example of, 25–26
    hospital as source of subjects for,
        59–60
    outline of, 22
    popularity of, 58
    schematic of design of, 56
    selection of population in, 59–60
    selection of sample in, 60–63
    sequential, 66–67
    time-order relationships in, 65–66
Currentness of information, 1, 4

Cutoff points in distribution, 136–37,
    141, 143, 189–91

Data. *See also* Statistical significance;
    Statistical tests.
    collection of, 111–25. *See also*
        Measurements.
    dredging of, 36
    pooling of, review articles and,
        246–48
Decision making:
    multivariate models and, 189–92
    prediction models and, 192
    risk-benefit balance and, 210–12
    sensitivity vs. specificity choice in,
        187–88
Descriptive studies, 15–18. *See also*
    Case series.
Design of study, 14–108
    basic, schematic of types of, 16
    case-control, 20–21, 23–24. *See also*
        Case-control studies.
    controlled trial, 18–19. *See also*
        Controlled trials; Experimental
        studies.
    cross-sectional, 22–23, 25–26. *See
        also* Cross-sectional studies.
    descriptive, 15–18
    experimental, 18–19, 26–27. *See also*
        Experimental studies.
    explanatory, 18–27
    follow-up, 21–22, 24–25. *See also*
        Follow-up studies.
    observational, 19–26
    prospective vs. retrospective, 29–30
    review article critique of, 245–46
    risk and, relative, 204–9
    terminology of, 14–15, 27–32
Diabetes mellitus:
    insulin infusion pumps for, 237–38
    retinopathy and, phenytoin and,
        88–89
Diagnosis:
    accuracy in, 83–85
    bias in, 38
    multiple tests and, 188–93
    regression models and, 173

Diagnosis (*cont.*):
　sensitivity, specificity and predictive
　　value in, 181–82, 187–88
　spectrum problem and, 193–94
　standards for, 194–96
　statistical significance and, 179–84
　uniform criteria for, data pooling
　　and, 247
Diet:
　blood pressure and, 158
　hemorrhoids and, 95
　vision and, 23–27, 204–7
Disclaimers, 255
Discriminant function analysis, 173,
　　174, 222
Discriminant scores, 189–91
Discussion sections, 7, 8, 255–56
Disease, normal distribution used to
　　define, 135–39
Distribution(s), 128–30
　central tendency in, 130–32
　chi-square test and, 164
　cutoff points in, 136–37, 141, 143,
　　189–91
　mean of, 130, 131
　　regression to, 140–43
　median of, 130–31
　　sampling variability and, 147
　mode of, 130–31
　　sampling variability and, 147
　normal (bell-shaped; Gaussian),
　　128, 134–39
　　disease defined by, 135–39
　　laboratory reporting methods
　　　and, 137–38
　percentiles in, 134
　　disease definition and, 136–37
　range of, 133
　skewed, 130, 131
　standard deviation in, 133
　　"abnormal" defined by, 137–39
　variability in, 132–34
Doctor Fox effect, 254
Dose-response relationship, 224–25
Double-blind trial, 122
Dropouts:
　in experimental study, 104–6

　in follow-up study, 70–73

Economic analyses, 196–98
　benefits and, 257
Editorials, 239–42
Educational programs:
　car seats for infants and, 119–20
　physician-ordered tests or
　　medications and, 120–21
Effectiveness of intervention, case
　　series and, 237–38
Efficacy, 83
Efficiency:
　in reading, 5–6
　of test, 183–84
Endometrial cancer:
　estrogen and, 210
　　biological plausibility and, 226–27
　　dose-response relationship and,
　　　224–25, 226
　smoking and, 210–11
End points, experimental study, 106–7
Entry criteria, experimental study,
　　83–85
Enzyme immunoassay, HIV screening
　　and, false positives and, 185–86
Estrogen:
　breast cancer and, 47
　contraception and, postcoital, 90–91
　endometrial cancer and, 210
　　biological plausibility and, 226–27
　　dose-response relationship of,
　　　224–25, 226
　fractures and, 256
Exact test, Fisher's, 165
Exercise, myocardial infarction and,
　　92–93, 103, 104
Expectation, observer, 116–18
Experimental studies, 18–19, 26–27,
　　78–108
　allocation of subjects in, 99–104
　attrition in, 104–6
　bias in, 94–97
　　allocation, 99–102
　classification methods for, 85–87
　cointervention and, 97
　compliance in, 94–97

controls in, 87–93
diagnostic accuracy and, 83–85
end points of, 106–7
entry criteria for, 83–85
generalizability of, 82, 83
historical note on, 78
intervention/treatment in, 93–99
  analysis by intention of, 105
  competing types of, 97
  compliance with, 94–97
  practicality of, 94
outline of, 19
placebo effect and, 88–89
population-selection problems,
  79–87
power of, 155–56
review article critique of, 245–46
stratification of subjects in, 102–4
terminology of, 32
Explanatory studies, 18–27
case-control, 20–21, 23–24. *See also*
  Case-control studies.
cross-sectional, 22–23, 25–26. *See*
  also Cross-sectional studies.
experimental, 18–19, 26–27. *See also*
  Experimental studies.
follow-up, 21–22, 24–25. *See also*
  Follow-up studies.
observational, 19–26
Explanatory trials, 83
Exposure data, case-control study and,
  45–50

False negatives, 184
False positives, 184
  HIV infection and, 185–86
  ROC curves and, 189–91
  sensitivity vs. specificity choice and,
    187–88
Feasibility, treatment, 237–38
Fetal heart rate, biased error and, 116–17
Fisher's exact test
Fluorescent antibody-coating bacterial
  assay, single-dose therapy of
  cystitis and, 80–81, 85–86
Follow-up studies, 21–22, 67–74
  bias in:

attrition, 71, 72
surveillance, 73–74
change in habits by subjects in, 73
example of, 24–25
loss of subjects in, 70–73
misuse of term for, 28
outline of, 21
prospective nature of, 29, 67–68
retrospective design and, 29
risk estimates and, 202
schematic of design of, 57
selection process in, 68–70
Fractures, estrogen and, 256
Frequency, relative risk and, 205–6
Frequency distribution, 128–30. *See*
  also Distribution.

Gauss's law, 128
Generalizability, 3–4
cholestyramine study and, 242
cross-sectional study population
  and, 59
diagnostic accuracy and, 83–85
experimental study population and,
  82, 83
follow-up study population and,
  69–70
statistical significance and, 146

Habit changes, follow-up subject, 73
Hair loss, cigar smoking and, 44,
  215–16
Hawthorne effect, 120–21
Health-care trials, 18, 32. *See also*
  Experimental studies.
Health services planning, 234–36
Heart murmurs, specificity vs.
  sensitivity choice in diagnosis of,
  187–88
Heart rate, fetal, biased error and,
  116–17
Heart studies:
anticoagulant therapy, 97, 101–2
aspirin trial, 82, 106
cholestyramine therapy, 241–42, 257
exercise, 92–93, 103, 104
lidocaine prophylaxis, 257

Heart studies (*cont.*):
  multiple risk factor intervention, 98
  personality type, 203–4
  pet ownership, 204, 217, 222
  response bias in, 64
  smoking, 209–10
  sugar consumption, 218–21
  sulfinpyrazone, 227–28
  timolol therapy, 104–5
  ventriculography, 194
Hedging, 255
Hemorrhoid therapy trial:
  classification problems and, 86
  cointerventions and, 97
  compliance in, 95–96
Historic controls, 91–92
HIV infection:
  convenience sampling and, 63
  false positive results and, 185–86
  population selection and, 60, 61
  sequential studies and, 66–67
Hospital:
  coffee consumption study in, 40, 242
  control subjects in, 39–40, 42, 242–43
  cross-sectional study population
    from, 59–60
  follow-up sample from, 69
  geriatrics unit of, 234–35
  multiple control groups and, 41
Human immunodeficiency virus. *See*
  HIV infection.
Hyperactivity, lead poisoning and,
  65–66
Hypercholesterolemia, cholestyramine
  therapy and, 241–42
Hypertension:
  alcohol consumption and, 30, 150
  compliance in therapy of, 98
  multiple risk factor intervention
    and, 98
  prevalence of, in adolescents,
    136–37, 141
  regression to the mean and, 140–42
Hypothesis generation, 36

Immunodeficiency virus. *See* HIV
  infection.

Inference, 146
Information, 1–2. *See also* Statistical
    significance; Statistical tests.
  biases in, 48
  currentness of, 1, 4
  primary vs. secondary sources of, 2
Intensive care patients, mortality
    prediction model for, 192
Intent in reading, 4–5
Interpretation, 127–229
  of causes, 214–29
  disagreement with authors on,
    256–57
  discussion/conclusions sections and,
    255–56
  of distributions, 127–44
  principle of, 12
  of risk, 201–13
  sensitivity, specificity, predictive
    value and, 178–99
  of statistical significance, 145–59
  statistical tests for, 161–77
  variability in, observer, 114–15
Interval data, 162
Intervention, 93–99. *See also*
    Treatment.
  analysis by intention of, 105
  competing types of, 97
  compliance and, 94–97
  evaluation of, 98–99
  practicality of, 94
Intervention trials, 18, 32. *See also*
    Experimental studies.
Interviewer:
  bias by, 48
  personality of, 118
Introduction section of study, 7–8
Investigator bias, 117–18

Journals, 4

Kappa value, 124

Laetrile therapy of cancer, 238–40
Lead poisoning, hyperactivity and,
  65–66
Letters to the editor, 239–43

new data in, 242–43
reliability of, 243
Linear relationships, correlation of, 169
Logistic regression, 173
Log linear models, 173
Loss of subjects, 70–73
  experimental studies and, 104–6
Lung cancer, smoking and, 38, 40,
    209–10
  bias testing and, 48
  consistency of evidence for, 228
  dose-response relationship of, 224,
    225

Mail, control selection by, 43
Management trial, 83
Matching, 43–45, 92–93
  confounding and, 215–16, 218
  excessive application of, 45
  risk and, relative, 207–8
"Materials and methods" section, 8
Mean, 130, 131
  regression to, 140–43
  standard deviation from, 133
  t test and, 167
Measurements, 111–25
  bias in, 116–22
    familiarity and, 121–22
    interviewer, 118
    investigator, 117–18
    subject, 118–22
  chance and, 124
  controlling errors in, 122–24
  distributions of, 128–30. *See also*
    Distributions.
  double-blind trial and, 122
  expectation and, 116–18
  familiarity with methods of, 121–22,
    141
  Hawthorne effect and, 120–21
  multiple, 143
  multiple data sources and, 123–24
  reliability of, 112
  repeated, 112, 121–22, 140–41
  second opinions and, 124
  standards and, 122–23
  systematic error in, 116–22

training in, 123
validity of, 112
variability in, 113–16, 140–42
Median, 130–31
  sampling variability and, 147
Memory, biased, 45–47
Mental health survey, interviewer bias
    and, 118
Metaanalysis, review articles and, 246–48
Methodology, 8
  review article critique of, 245–46
  concentration on, 11–12
Misclassification, 140–42
  diagnostic technique evaluation and,
    180–81
  discriminant scores and, 189
  experimental study and, 83–85
  sensitivity vs. specificity choice in,
    187–88
Mode, 130–31
  sampling variability and, 147
Multicenter trial, 81
Multiple control groups, 41–42
Multiple risk factor intervention trial,
    98
Multiple sclerosis, animal contact and,
    206–9
Multiple tests, 188–93
Multivariate regression techniques,
    173–76, 189–92
  confounding and, 221–22
Myocardial infarction:
  anticoagulant therapy and, 97, 101–2
  aspirin in prevention of, 82, 106
  diagnostic standard for, 196
  exercise and, 92–93, 103, 104
  sugar consumption and, 219
  sulfinpyrazone and, 227–28
  timolol and, 104–5

Natural history of disease, 232–34
Negative test, 182
  false, 184
Nested case-control study, 48–50
Nominal data, 161
  chi-square test and, 165–66
Noncompliance, 94–97

Normality (in distribution), 128,
134–39
disease defined by, 135–39
laboratory reporting methods and,
137–38
Null hypothesis, 148–49
chi-square test and, 164
confidence interval and, 157
errors in testing, 154–56
failure to reject, 152–54
t test and, 167

Obfuscation, 253–54
Objectivity, 48, 118. *See also* Bias.
Observational studies, 19–26
case-control, 20–21, 23–24. *See also*
Case-control studies.
cross-sectional, 22–23, 25–26. *See
also* Cross-sectional studies.
follow-up, 21–22, 24–25. *See also*
Follow-up studies.
Observer(s):
expectations of, 116–18
Hawthorne effect and, 120–21
multiple, 123–24
personality of, 118
training of, 123
variability in, 113–16
Odds, relative, 205–9
Odds ratio, 205–9
Ordinal data, 162
chi-square test and, 165
Overmatching, 45

p value, 149–50
chi-square test and, 164
confidence interval and, 156–57
correlation coefficient and, 169
sample size and, 150, 153
t test and, 167
Pancreatic cancer, coffee consumption
and, 39–40
letters to the editor on, 242–43
Participation bias, 63–65
"Patients and methods" section, 8
Pearson correlation coefficient, 169,
171

Percentiles, 134
disease definition and, 136–37
Pet ownership, heart disease and, 204,
217, 222
Pharyngitis:
streptococcal, prediction models for,
192, 196–97
tonsillectomy and, 141–43
Physicians:
as experimental study subjects
(aspirin-heart disease study),
82, 106
Hawthorne effect and, 120–21
Placebo effect, 88–89
Planning, health services, 234–36
Pooling of data, 246–48
Population(s), 17–18, 22
cases chosen in, 36–38
chi-square test of, 164
clinic based study, 69–70
controls in, 39
multiple, 41
cross-sectional study, 59–60
experimental study, 79–87
follow-up study, 68–70
"general," 39
HIV seroprevalence and, 60, 61
nested case-control study and, 48–50
prospective design and, 29
risk, 202
relative, 204–5
spectrum problem and, 193–94
t test of, 167–68
Positive test, 182
false. *See* False positives.
pretest probability and, 184–85
standards and, 195
Posterior probability, 184–86
Posttest probability, 184–86
Power:
experimental (statistical), 155–56
of metaanalysis (data pooling), 246
Practicality of treatment, 94
Prediction models:
cost considerations and, 197
mortality, intensive care patients
and, 192

prevalence and, 192–93
regression techniques and, 173,
174–75
streptococcal pharyngitis and, 192,
196–97
Predictive value, 181–83, 188
definition of, 182
prevalence and, 184–85
standards and, 195
statistical significance and, 179–84
Pregnancy:
DES studies and, 91–92
postcoital contraceptive study and,
90–91
risk of, 211
smoking and alcohol consumption in,
febrile seizures in infant related
to, 37, 43
Pretest, bias and, 122
Pretest probability, 184–86
Prevalence, 184–86
prediction models and, 192–93
Prevalence studies, 22–23. *See also*
Cross-sectional studies.
Primary sources, 2
Prior probability, 184–86
Probability:
chi-square test and, 164
Fisher's exact test and, 165
p value and, 149
posttest (posterior), 184–86
pretest (prior), 184–86
Prospective study, 29–30

Qualifying words or phrases, 255

Radiographs, variability in
interpretation of, 114–15
Radionuclide ventriculography, 194
Random allocation, 99, 100
Random sampling, 61
Range of distribution, 133
Rare disease, case-control design and,
35
Ratio data, 162
Readability, 254
Reasons for reading, 4–6

Recall, selective (biased), 45–47
Receiver-operating characteristic
curve, 189–91
References, 8–9
Referral center:
cross-sectional study population
from, 59–60
follow-up sample from, 69
multiple controls and, 41
Regression analysis, 171–76
multivariate, 173–76, 189–92
confounding and, 221–22
Regression to the mean, 140–43
Relative risk, 203–9
study design and, 204–9
Reliability of measurements, 112
Reporting bias, 38
Reproducibility, 112
Research bias, 47–48
Research hypothesis, 148
Response bias, 47, 50, 63–65
Results section, 8, 255
Retrospective study, 29–30
Reviews, 243–48
content, 243
metaanalysis (data pooling) in,
246–48
methodological critique in, 245–46
selection process used for, 244
Reye's syndrome, 38–39, 41–42
Risk, 201–13
attributable, 209–10
balancing, 210–12
case-control studies and, 204–9
confidence interval and, 208–9
population-based studies and,
204–5
ratios of, 203, 205–8
confounding and, 215–16
relative, 203–9
vs. attributable risk, 209–10
study design and, 204–9
statements of, 202
ROC curve, 189–91

Salicylates, Reye's syndrome and,
41–42

Sampling:
  biased, 61, 62
    in case-control study, 37, 38
  case-control study, 36–38
  case definition and, 38–39
  change and, 215
  community controls and, 42–43
  convenience, 61, 63
  cross-sectional study, 60–63
  follow-up study, 69
  inferences and, 146
  laissez-faire, 61
  random, 61
  risk ratios and, 208
  sequential studies and, 66
  size of, 155, 156
    metaanalysis (data pooling) and, 246
    p value and, 150, 153
  systematic, 61
  variability in, statistical significance and, 147–48, 153
Scanning (of articles), 10–11
Screening:
  breast cancer, 195
  sensitivity vs. specificity choice in, 187–88
Secondary sources, 2
Seizures, febrile, in children:
  follow-up study and, 68–69
  maternal smoking and alcohol consumption and, 37, 43
Selection:
  biased:
    allocation and, 99, 101, 102
    spectrum problem and, 194
  of cases, in case-control study, 36–39
  of controls:
    in case-control study, 39–40
    in experimental study, 87–93
  population:
    in cross-sectional study, 59–60
    in experimental study, 79–87
    in follow-up study, 68–70
    spectrum problem and, 193–94
  random, 61

review article, 244
sample. See also Sampling.
  in cross-sectional study, 60–63
Selective recall, 45–47
Selectivity in reading, 9–10
Self-criticism, 255–56
Sensitivity, 181–88
  choice of specificity vs., 187–88
  cost considerations and, 197
  definition of, 182
  prevalence and, 184–86
  receiver-operated characteristic (ROC) curve, 189–91
  spectrum problem and, 193–94
  standards and, 195–96
  summary questions on, 198
Sequential studies, cross-sectional, 66–67
Serology, HIV, 61
  false positives and, 185–86
  sequential studies and, 67
Sickle cell anemia, overmatching and, 45
SIDS, 46–47
Significance testing. See Statistical significance.
Single-dose vs. multidose therapy of urinary tract infections, 80–81, 153–54
  classification and, 85–86
  confidence interval and, 157
  metaanalysis (data pooling) and, 246–48
Smoking:
  cigar, baldness and, 44, 215–16
  endometrial cancer and, 210–11
  heart disease and, 209–10
    sugar consumption and, 219–21
  lung cancer and, 38, 40, 209–10
    bias testing and, 48
    consistency of evidence for, 228
    dose-response relationship of, 224, 225
  maternal, febrile seizures in infant and, 37, 43
  multiple risk factor intervention and, 98

risk and, relative vs. attributable, 209–10
sugar (sucrose) consumption and, 218–21
Social desirability bias, 119–20
Specificity, 181–88
  choice of sensitivity vs., 187–88
  definition of, 182
  prevalence and, 184–86
  receiver-operating characteristic (ROC) curve, 189–91
  spectrum problem and, 193–94
  summary questions on, 198
Spectrum (of disease course), 193–94
Standard deviation, 133
  "abnormal" defined by, 137–39
Standards, 194–96
  measurement and, 122–23
Statistical significance, 145–59
  alpha error and, 154, 155
  beta (type II) errors and, 154–56, 166
  bias and, 158–59
  clinical impact and, 150–52
  confidence intervals and, 156–57
  diagnostic technique and, 179–84
  inference and, 146
  null hypothesis and, 148–49
    errors in testing, 154–56
    failure to reject, 152–54
  p value and, 149–50. *See also* p value.
  size of sample and, 150, 153
  power of study and, 155–56
  relevance of, 157–59
  sampling variability and, 147–48, 153
Statistical tests, 161–77
  categorical data and, 164–66
  chi-square, 164–65
  continuous data and, 162, 166–68
  correlation, 169–71
  Fisher's exact, 165
  interval data and, 162
  nominal data and, 161
  ordinal data and, 162
  ratio data and, 162
  regression analysis, 171–76
  t (Student's), 166–68

Stepwise multiple regression, 173
Stratification of subjects, 102–4
  control-table method of, 218–21
Streptococcal pharyngitis, prediction models for, 192, 196–97
Stroke, carotid artery surgery and, 105–6
Structure of article, 6–9
  scanning and, 11
Student's t test, 166–68
Study design. *See* Design of study.
Subheadings, 11
Subjects. *See also* Case; Population.
  allocation of, 99–104
  alternation of, 88–89
  bias from, 45–47, 118–22
  change in habits of, 73
  classification of. *See also* Classification.
    technical procedures and, 85–87
  comparison. *See* Controls.
  cooperation of, 63–65
  crossover of, 88–89
  cross-sectional study, 59–63
  experimental study, 79–87
  loss of, 70–73
    in experimental study, 104–6
  matching of. *See* Matching.
  stratification of, 102–4
    control-table method of, 218–21
Sugar consumption, heart disease and, 218–21
Summary, 6–7
Surveillance bias, 73–74
Sweetener's, artificial:
  bladder cancer and, 225, 226, 228
  neurological symptoms and, 89–90
Systematic error, 116–22
Systematic sampling, 61

t test, 166–68
Tampons, toxic shock syndrome and, 37–38, 202, 239–41
Technical procedures, classification of subjects and, 85–87
Telephone, control selection by, 41, 43

Terminology of study design, 14–15, 27–32
  tabulation of, 16, 31
Tests:
  efficiency of, 183–84
  multiple, 188–93
  sensitivity, specificity, and predictive value of, 181–83. *See also* Predictive value; Sensitivity; Specificity.
  standards for, 194–96
  statistical. *See* Statistical tests.
Therapy. *See* Treatment.
Time-order relationships, 65–66
Toxic shock syndrome, 37–38, 202, 239–41
Training:
  observer, 123
Treatment, 93–99
  analysis by intention of, 105
  case series and, 236–39
  competing types of, 97
  compliance with, 94–97
  effectiveness of, 238–39
  evaluation of, 98–99
  feasibility of, 237–38
  null hypothesis and. *See* Null hypothesis.
  practicality of, 94
  regression models and, 173
  similar regimens of, data pooling and, 247
  single-dose vs. multidose, 80–81, 85–86, 153–54, 157, 246–48
Type I error, 154, 155
Type II error, 154–56, 166

metaanalysis (data pooling) and, 246, 248

Urinary bladder, cancer of, artificial sweeteners and, 225, 226, 228
Urinary tract infection:
  amoxicillin for, 80–81, 85–86, 153–54
  in schoolgirls, 28, 131–32
  single-dose vs. multidose therapy for, 80–81, 153–54
  classification and, 85–86
  confidence interval and, 157
  metaanalysis (data pooling) and, 246–48
"Usual," concept of, 139

Validity, 3–4
  external, 3–4. *See also* Generalizability.
  case series and, 236
  internal, 3
    entry criteria and, 83
    experimental study population and, 82, 83
  measurement, 112
  reproducibility and, 112
Variability:
  in distribution, 132–34
  in measurements, 113–16, 140–42
  sampling, statistical significance and, 147–48, 153
Variance, 176

Washout period, 89
Writing skills, 253–55